YOGA AND DIET
FOR WEIGHT LOSS

Bijoylaxmi Hota is a noted Integrated Yoga Therapist whose books sell internationally. She gives as much importance to diet as to yoga, since diet plays a major role in one's health. With forty years of experience, Hota has cured ailments, such as acidity, asthma, backache, diabetes, bronchitis, hypertension, tumour and many more, with her brand of Integrated Yoga. She has written nine books on yoga and diet, including the bestseller *Yoga for Busy People*.

She lives in Delhi.

YOGA AND DIET
FOR WEIGHT LOSS

by Bijoylaxmi Hota

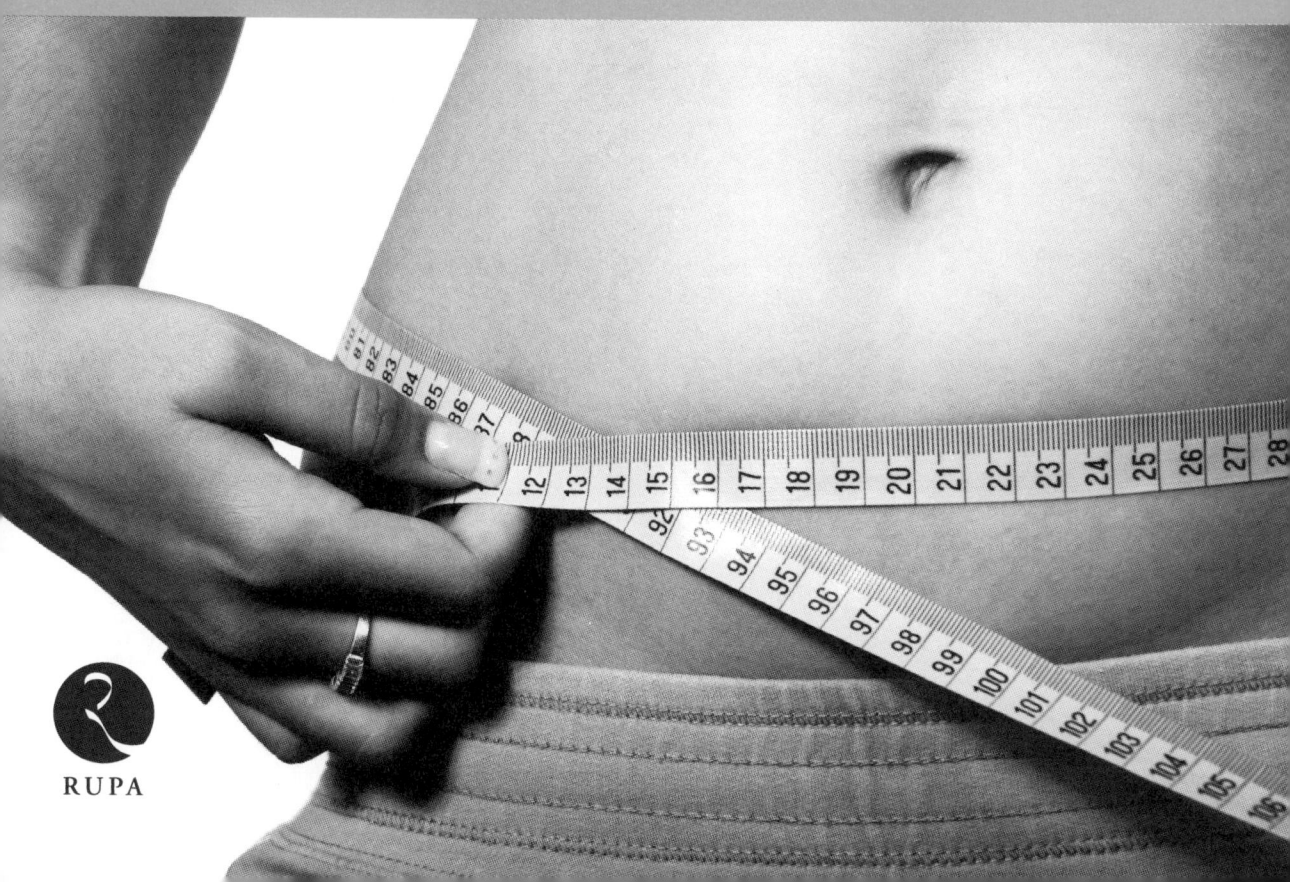

RUPA

Published by
Rupa Publications India Pvt. Ltd 2019
7/16, Ansari Road, Daryaganj
New Delhi 110002

Sales centres:
Allahabad Bengaluru Chennai
Hyderabad Jaipur Kathmandu
Kolkata Mumbai

Copyright © Bijoylaxmi Hota 2019
Design & Illustrations © Ishtihaar.com 2019

While every effort has been made to verify the authenticity of the information contained in this book, it is not intended as a substitute for medical consultation with a physician. Yoga should be learned directly from an expert to avoid risks. The publisher and the author are in no way liable for the use of the information contained in this book.

All rights reserved.

No part of this publication may be reproduced, transmitted, or stored in a retrieval system, in any form or by any means, electronic, mechanical, photocopying, recording or otherwise, without the prior permission of the publisher.

ISBN: 978-93-5333-486-4

First impression 2019

10 9 8 7 6 5 4 3 2 1

The moral right of the author has been asserted.

Printed by Excel Printers Pvt. Ltd. New Delhi

This book is sold subject to the condition that it shall not, by way of trade or otherwise, be lent, resold, hired out, or otherwise circulated, without the publisher's prior consent, in any form of binding or cover other than that in which it is published.

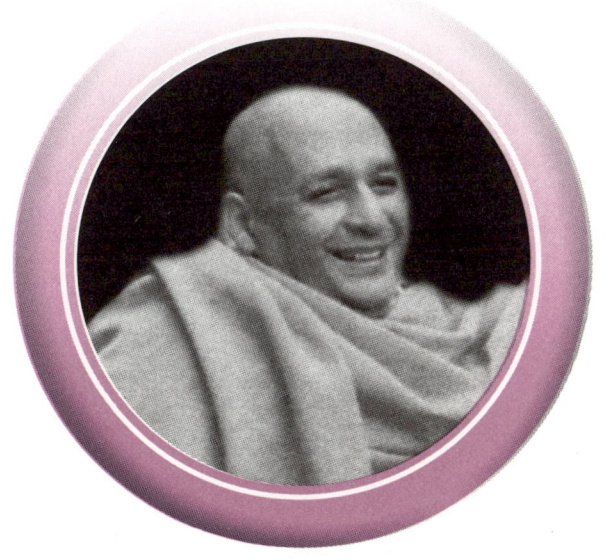

With the blessings of my Guru and Guide
Parmahamsa Swami Sri Satyananda Sarswati

Contents

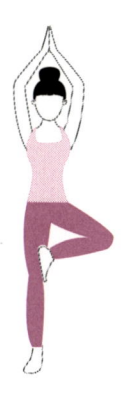

The Key	8
Right Choice	16
Ridding the Evil	24
A Gentle Start	36
Faster Metabolism	46
Dynamic Asanas	56
Prana Enhancer	68
Sleep to Succeed	78
Via the Mind	86
Tackling Depression	92
Food Facts	104
Slimming Recipes	116
Important Tips	130

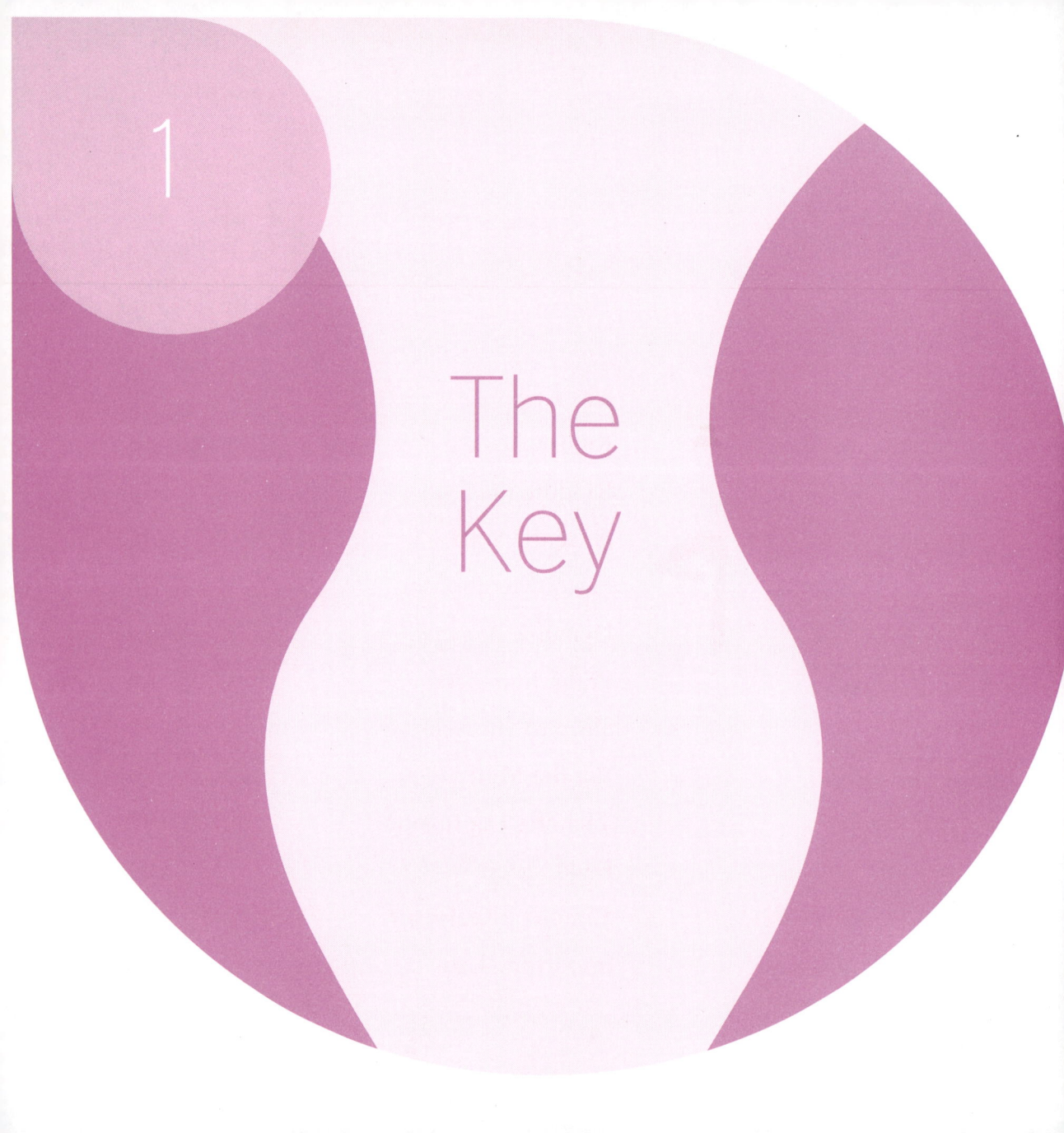

1 The Key

The Key

If you are trying to lose weight, which most probably you are, this is the right book for you. Unlike most other weight loss programmes, which are partial and superficial in their approach, the methods contained in this book deal with the deeper and more subtle aspects of a human being and root out the core causes.

At the onset, it will do you well to remember one thing—slimming is not just about what you eat, how much you eat, how much you exercise or what form of exercise you do. These are important. But more importantly, it is how fast your body utilizes your food. In other words, how efficient is your metabolism. In obese people, it is very sluggish while slim people have faster metabolism. You must have seen some people who have to struggle hard to keep their weight from going down. They gorge on all kinds of high-calorie foods such as butter, cream, cakes and cookies, and yet are painfully thin. It is because their body uses up every calorie they put into their mouths. Although it is a health hazard and should not be aimed for, it shows to what extreme the human metabolism can rise. Hence, the target should be to hasten the process and make it so fast that without being a clinical problem, it can burn all your extra calories quickly. And that is exactly what you are going to learn.

To alter the body's tendencies, we need to understand how the body works. We do not realize that every physical function is the result of a highly complex process. Even a simple action such as blinking of the eyes is not as simple as it seems. It involves many body parts such as the nerves to carry the message to and from the brain, the brain to analyse the message and send out its instructions, the blood vessels to supply blood for the job, and the muscles of the eyelids that have to shut and open. Not just the body but, even the 'inner intelligence' gets involved in all physical functions, as the body cannot do anything independently—it just follows the mind's orders. The brain's job is only to execute them by coordinating with the various parts of the body.

Metabolism is a far complex process than the blinking of the eyes. It is a major systemic function that involves a still larger number of body parts. Apart from the body and its inner intelligence, the process is greatly influenced by our emotions. We all know how our saliva secretion stops and our mouths dry up when we are frightened, or how our hunger disappears when we are depressed. It is only when our emotions are balanced that the body functions normally. That is why dealing with weight gain on a purely physical level is not very successful. It may seem otherwise for a while, but soon the intelligence creates such physical conditions that the same method becomes ineffective after some time. Therefore, the mind and the psyche have to be first taken care of for the desired result.

Sometimes, in spite of conducive physical conditions and the right instructions, the body parts do not carry out the orders. It is not because of any deliberate disobedience on their part, but simply because they do not have the strength to perform the task, which is the result of the lack of necessary nourishments. Nourishments does not mean only vitamins and minerals but also the subtle bio energy called *Prana*.

Prana is the vital force that is essential to life. It is such an important substance that one can live without food, water and oxygen for sometime—as Yogis have often done—but not without *prana* . As long as *prana* remains in the body, we live and the moment it leaves us, we die. And in life no body cell can function without this energy, the more they have, better is their health and efficiency. Therefore, it is necessary to increase its amount in the body.

Prana enters the body from the atmosphere and plys in special energy channels called *nadis*. There are 72,000 *nadis* in our body to carry this vital force to every body tissue. To regulate the flow of *prana* in the *nadis*, there are many energy centres called *chakras*. These *chakra's* store *prana* and send out the required amount to its surrounding body parts as and when necessary. Due to various reasons, a blockage may occur in the *nadis* and make a *chakra* sluggish. Then, the body parts in its surrounding area do not get enough *prana* to do their job correctly. Consequently, their functions go haywire and health problems manifest.

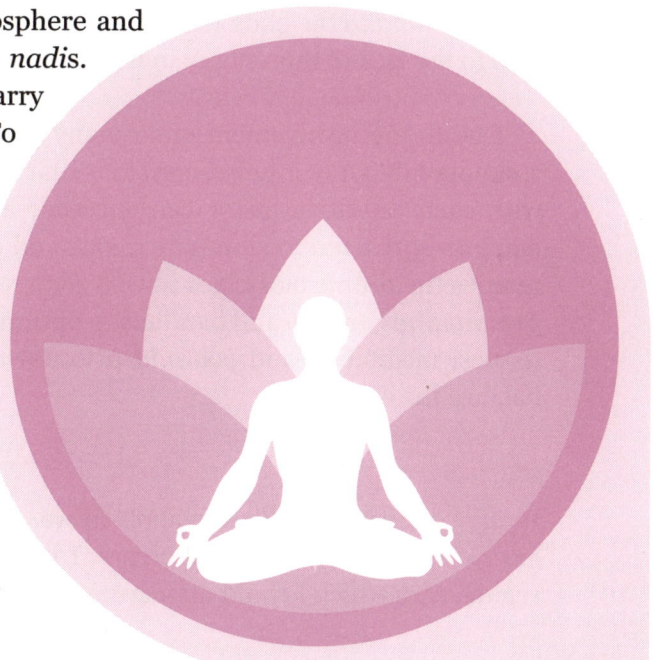

According to Yoga, trouble starts mostly in the mind. It maintains that when the mind is tense, nurtures negative emotions, or thinks too much about a subject, the *prana* is directed more to the *ida nadi*—meant to energize all mental work—leaving less *prana* for the Pingala nadi, which supplies energy to the body tissues for physical activities. This imbalance causes blockages.

Apart from the mental stress, toxins and excessive humour can also obstruct the flow of *prana* to the body tissues. Also, one's surrounding with inadequate *prana* can lead to the lack of this energy in the body.

Due to the involvement of so many factors in metabolism, setting it right is not a simple job. Only a holistic system that has the techniques to simultaneously deal with each causative factor can succeed; and Integrated Yoga is such a system. It employs *satkarma* to eliminate toxins and excess humours from the body; *asana*s to remove the *pranic* blockages as well as to rectify the defects in the glands and organs; *pranayama*s, mudra and bandhas to optimize *prana* and ensure its correct flow to the tissues; meditation and *yoganidra* to de-stress the mind; and music and mantra to balance the emotions.

My discovery and experience

In my younger days, my metabolism was very slow and I used to put on weight very easily. After many trials and errors, I had learned a dietary pattern and an exercise regime with which I could manage to keep my weight under control till I took steroids for a health problem. Within a short period, I put on as much as thirty kilos. It was the worst phase of my life. Not only was I self-conscious and felt uncomfortable all the time, people made me feel worse with their words and look of pity, sympathy, advice and even derision. As the obvious, I was terribly stressed, unhappy, angry and frustrated. That must have made my problem still worse, as these negative emotions are major factors that disturb the smooth functioning of the system. And to add to the woes, I kept failing in my repeated attempts to lose weight.

Now I know why I was not successful in my endeavour. Like most other overweight people, my methods were all wrong. I too only focussed on my body. I starved, jogged and exercised, it wouldn't yield much result. Although I did lose some weight sometimes, but never enough compared to the effort and pain I had been going through. After a while, I stopped trying altogether and started eating everything that an overweight person shouldn't.

I loathe to think what that must have done to my system. The blood must have gotten slushier, making it harder for the heart to push the thick fluid into my body tissues, that too, to so many more of them now. Same must have happened with the pancreas, which had to secrete so much more insulin to process that large amount of food. No wonder diabetes, high blood pressure and heart attacks are so common in obese people. Not just these two organs but other parts suffer as well when the body bloats. The delicate nerve cells get chafed by the excessive fat causing a depression in the nervous system, which can lead to mental depression. Sleep apnea is yet another common problem, and with disturbed sleep, one's mood, appearance and energy level are adversely affected. Thus, physically, mentally, emotionally and aesthetically, obesity can wreck a person completely.

Perhaps that was the reason why I was so unhealthy those days. I accumulated ailments after ailments. They were getting worse by the day, and were not responding to any treatment—conventional or otherwise. How could they, when the root cause was left untouched? Luckily for me, my mother, who had cured her diabetes with yoga in the local yogashram, suggested that I go and stay there for some time and get myself treated. I decided to do that as the last resort.

Yoga's effect on me was quick and magical. In just fifteen days in the ashram, most of my problems had disappeared. Although my steroid's effects had waned by then and I was not as grossly overweight, whatever extra weight I still had, vanished, that too with much more food than I used to have earlier. I was thrilled. Finally, I had found the perfect formula to stay slim without bothering much about food. All I needed to do was to practise regularly and religiously the yogic techniques meant to speed up the body's metabolism. And till date, when I am more than seventy years old, it has never disappointed me.

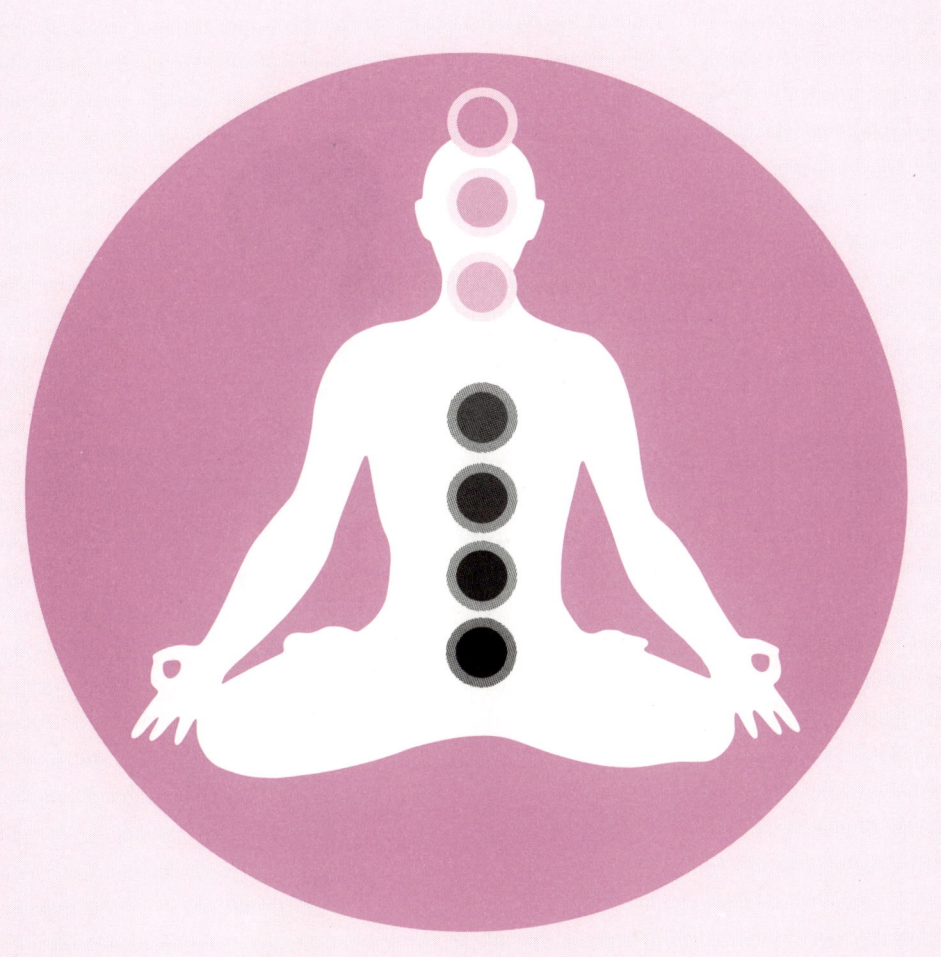

2

Right Choice

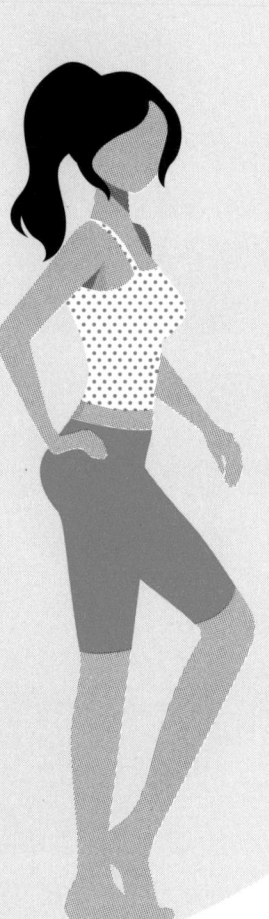

Right Choice

Weight watchers, who are tempted to combine yoga with other slimming methods for better results, should keep in mind that yoga with the right food is a complete and effective treatment. It does not need other systems to enhance its efficacy. Besides, the other popular methods prevalent today can have undesirable consequences.

Extreme low-calorie diet: This is the most common method every weight watcher follows. It may seem the ideal way to keep the weight down, but surprisingly researchers have not found many evidence that all small eaters are thinner than all big eaters. In a research, 40 women took 1,500 calories a day while another 40 women consumed 2,400 calories per day. At the end of the research period, the small eaters weighed 9 pounds more than the big eaters. They explain it as the famine phenomenon. It implies that when not enough food is consumed, the body perceives it as a famine situation, and as a self-preservation measure, it slows down the metabolic rate to survive longer. Worse is, it does not take long for that to happen. It has been seen that within a day or two, the metabolic rate can drop by 15 to 30 per cent. This means the

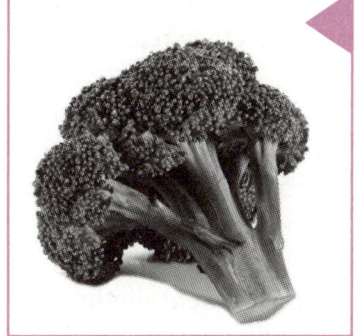

dieter has to reduce the calorie intake further to achieve the goal, which becomes a health risk. People with a very low-calorie diet can develop various problems such as low blood-pressure, elevated cholesterol, high uric acid, anaemia, gallstone, nausea, weakness and severe headaches.

Even if one loses weight through a very low calorie diet, the lost weight always comes back after a while, and invariably with a few extra kilos. A study conducted by Dr Allen King on 500 of his patients who were given 500 to 1,000 calories a day revealed that in six months they lost 50 pounds, and in three years after that, the average gain was 60 pounds. Unfortunately, dieters lose both muscles and fat tissues while they are dieting, but when they regain, it is mostly fat that comes back.

Some scientists say that dieting itself can cause obesity. They have found that men with a low-calorie diet, the thyroid hormone decreases by 28.3 per cent in six weeks. Thyroid Stimulating Hormone (TSH), which stimulates the secretion of the thyroid hormone, is also found depressed. Naturally, the outcome is weight gain.

Intermittent dieting is still worse. After analysing 3,000 cases, researchers found that a fluctuating weight had a 75 per cent greater risk of dying from heart diseases. And for men with yo-yo diet, the risk was as high as 93 per cent. Besides, during each phase of dieting, the metabolic rate is slower than the previous phase, and it takes longer for it to recover. So weight is gained more and more rapidly, and the same low-calorie diet becomes more and more ineffective after each phase.

The protein rich diet Favoured by most modern dieticians, this is a very popular slimming method. As the name suggests, in this diet, people need to increase their protein intake considerably and decrease their carbohydrates to the barest minimum. As protein is harder to digest than other nutrients, the body has to now spend a lot more calories than it usually does to supply the extra energy to the digestive system, and the result is weight loss.

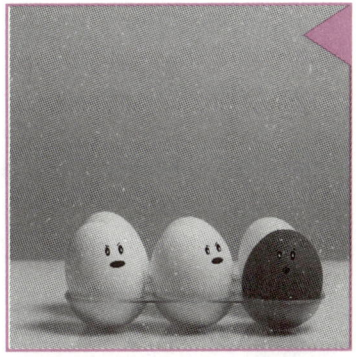

But in this dietary pattern, the system can suffer badly, because the end product of protein metabolism is uric acid, and a high level of this acid in the blood is extremely harmful. First, it puts undue strain on the kidneys and affects their efficiency. As the kidneys are the body's detoxifying organs, if they do not do their job well, the system can get slowly and steadily poisoned. Furthermore, once these vital organs are adversely affected, it is extremely difficult to reverse their conditions. In the long run, this could lead to a more toxic body and eventually kidney failure. Secondly, too much protein can harden the blood vessels putting our health and life at a great risk, as a stiff blood vessel can rupture easily causing a stroke. And lastly, an acidic body is ideal for the development of serious ailments such as cancer. An acidic body also attracts and holds on to all kinds of infections. I know of a girl who followed a protein rich diet and lost a lot of weight. However, she soon developed a vaginal infection that just would not go away even with medication. She continued to suffer severe burning through the day and night for months till she switched over to an alkaline diet and got better.

Too much salad It is a common belief that salads being of very low calorie, facilitates weight loss. Wrong! I met an obese lady who virtually lived on salads but was not losing any weight. The reason being–too much raw vegetables can inhibit our thyroxin production, and low thyroxin means slower metabolism and weight gain.

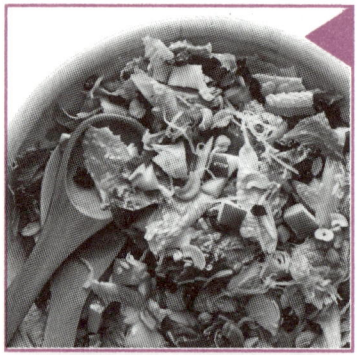

Mono diet This is a strange weight loss method, where you are allowed to eat only one kind of food per day. You can choose any food you want. So if it is banana, you eat only bananas the whole day; if it is 'gulab jamun' you have only 'gulab jamuns' that day. A diet like that is bound to lead to nutritional deficiencies, and deficiencies of certain nutrients, especially iron and calcium, can cause weight gain, because fat can be burned only in the presence of these two minerals. Nutritional deficiencies can also affect one's appearance adversely. I was told about a girl who was following this diet pattern. She lost her weight and also lost a lot of her hair; her muscles sagged, and her skin looked dull.

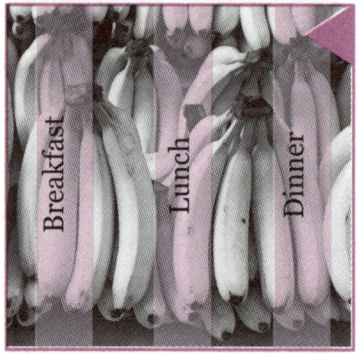

Frequent eating Another diet programme that has emerged these days is, eating every two hours. People claim to have lost a lot of weight through this method, but there is no evidence that this method actually works. According to an article published in 2010 in the *British Journal of Nutrition*, a study was conducted on the effect of six meals verses three in two groups of obese adults with the same calorie intake. The researchers found no difference in their weight loss after eight weeks of study. Critics say that the fat loss is not due to frequent eating, but the total calorie reduction.

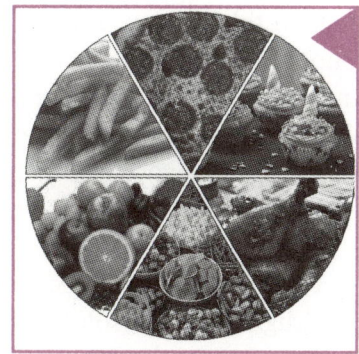

In frequent eating the constant stimulation of acidic gastric juices can cause acidity of the blood, which has been explained as a dangerous condition. It also harms the digestive system, as in this pattern, the digestive organs have to work almost continuously and no body part can remain healthy without adequate rest. There should be three to five hours gap between meals to give proper rest to the stomach.

Stomach stapling This is a surgical procedure where the stomach is stapled to decrease its inner space making it impossible to hold much food. People who find it difficult to restrict their food intake, happily turn to this

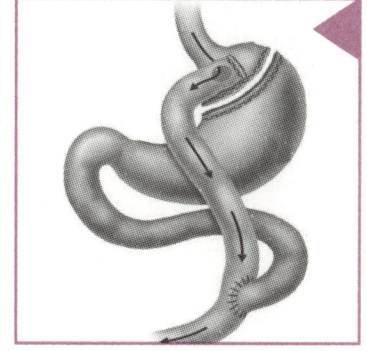

method taking it as an ideal means to solve their problem. A study, during a five year follow-up, showed that, of the 104 people who had resorted to this surgery, five died and there were health complications in the rest, such as gastric perforation, venous thrombosis, pulmonary embolism and various infections. What is disappointing is that, the lost weight returned even with the staple.

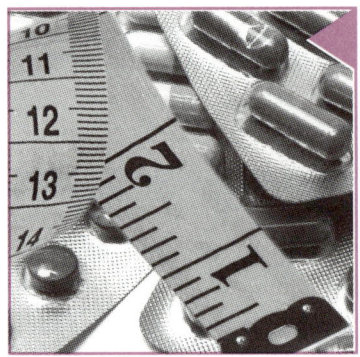

Diet pills This is perhaps the worst of them all, as drugs are no solution for any health problem. Rather, they harm the system as they are artificial, and everything unnatural is unwelcome by the body. They pollute the blood, weaken the organs and disturb the inner functioning. And, there are a number of instances where even youngsters in their teens have died due to ravaged livers caused by these pills.

Yoga, on the other hand, is an ancient science that has proved its efficacy and safety over centuries. It understands the human system perfectly and proceeds to rectify its defects in a systematic manner.

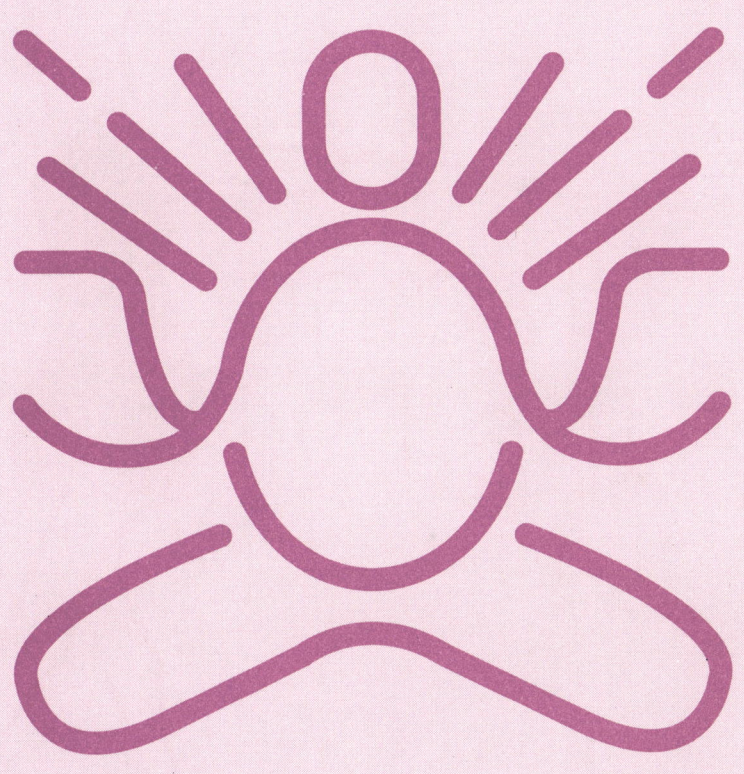

2
Ridding the Evil

Ridding the Evil

Yogic treatment starts with ridding the system of chemicals and other toxins. In our daily life, we consume a lot of chemicals in the form of drugs and food that has pesticides, insecticides, preservatives, food additives and food colourings. The water and air too have many chemicals. As long as these toxins are present in the body, perfect health of any body part is not possible. Because these foreign matters not only make the system toxic, they too can create *pranic* blockages. In such a toxic condition, even clearing the *pranic* blockages has little value. Soon, they are bound to reappear. Furthermore, chemicals are artificial and our body does not like anything that is not natural. It tries its best to get rid of them putting extra load on the liver and the kidneys. Sometimes more humuors are produced to trap them.

As one grows older, the situation becomes worse. Toxins continue to pile up while the body gets progressively weaker, and the metabolism becomes more sluggish. Which is why people over forty are seen to gain weight even with much less than a thousand calories.

For all these reasons, yoga gives maximum importance to detoxification. For that purpose, it contains six cleansing techniques called *satkarma*. In fact, initially *Hatha Yoga*—the yoga of the body—comprised only these practices. *Asana*s and *pranayama*s, which are now considered as the only Yoga by most people, were added much later.

Among all the *satkarmas*, Guru Shankha Prakshyalan is the most important one. This practice not only removes all unwanted matters from the body, it is also a great reviver of the system. The practice involves drinking a large amount of water, doing specific *asana*s and evacuating the bowel. The process is continued till the intestine is completely empty. Not only the entire digestive tract is washed thoroughly, the water circulating over the body draws the stored toxins from the tissues and throws them out. Thus, the whole body is made scrupulously clean within a few hours, and a smooth *pranic* flow is re-established.

After the cleansing is done, one is required to lie down quietly for forty-five minutes. During that period, there is no food in the system to be metabolized, meaning, there is no work for the thyroid. For once, it gets complete rest—a kind it can never get by any other means. Such total rest along with the increased *prana*, gives this gland a perfect chance to heal and rejuvenate itself. It has been seen that even the most sluggish thyroid starts working efficiently after *Guru Shankha Prakshyalana*. The effect is felt within a day or two when the appetite increases greatly, food is digested in no time, and the body fat starts melting. People generally lose 3 kg to 4 kg in three to four weeks after this practice. I have myself seen some practitioners losing even 10 kg to 12 kg in two months.

Ideally, *Guru Shankha Prakshyalana* should be done once a year in a pure and peaceful surrounding away from home. Although it is not repeated for a year, if the thyroid is too sluggish for too long, it can be done again after six months. However, it should be done only under expert supervision, as it has many rules and regulations which have to be followed strictly. Overlooking any point, no matter how insignificant it might seem, can negate its effects. The disregard can even cause irreversible damage to the system. Therefore, if all the facilities are not available, you should never attempt this practice. Instead, you could do its minor version called *Laghoo Shankha Prakshyalana.*

Although not as powerful as the major one, when practised daily over a period, *Laghoo Shankha Prakshyalan* can give almost the same benefits. The best part about this practice is, unlike *Guru Shankha Prakshyalan*, it requires no restrictions whatsoever. Anybody can do it anytime and anywhere. Not only for detoxification, but for slimming too this is a great practice. Because it makes the blood sugar fall immediately, forcing the body to melt the stored fat for quick energy resulting in weight loss.

The technique *(To be done first thing in the morning.)*

- Heat six glasses of water (it should be hot, but not so much that you can't drink it quickly.)
- Add one and a half spoon of salt in the water and mix it well. Quickly drink two glasses of this water and then practice the following *asanas*:

Tadasana

- Stand straight.
- Interlock your fingers and place them on your head.
- Inhaling, lift your heels and stretch your arms above you (hands turned outwards).
- Turn your face up to look at the hands.
- Exhaling, return to the starting position by banging your heels down.
- Practise 8 times.

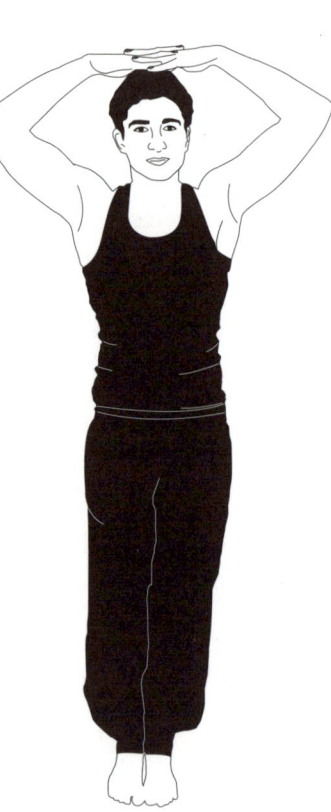
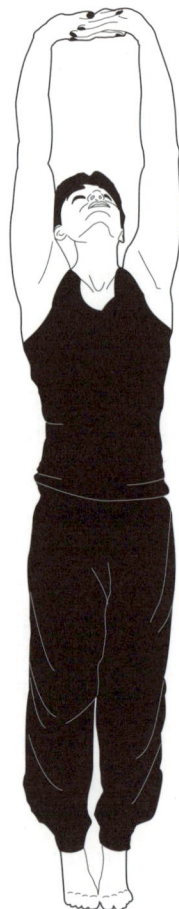

Triyak Tadasana

- Stand with fingers interlocked.
- Stretch your arms above you with your palms out and move your legs apart.
- Take a deep breath.
- Exhaling, bend to your left.
- Inhaling, return to the starting position.
- Exhaling, bend to your right.
- Inhaling, return to the starting position.
- Repeat 4 times.

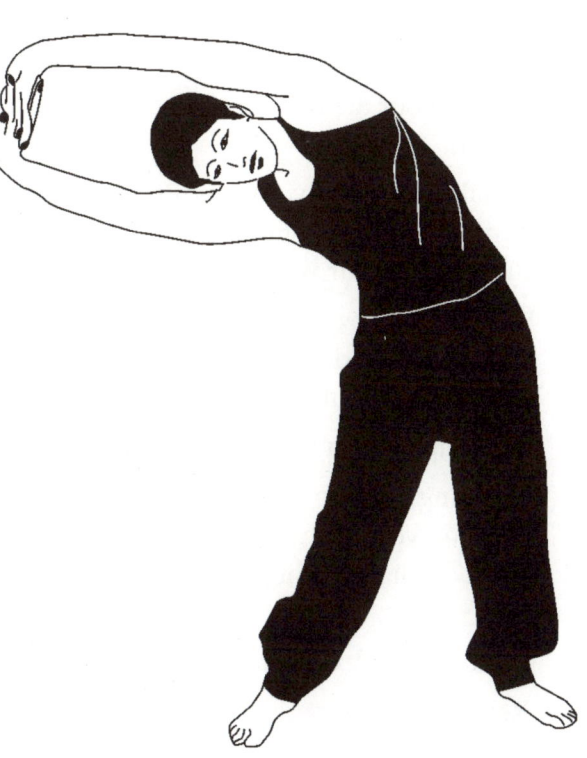

KATI CHAKRASANA

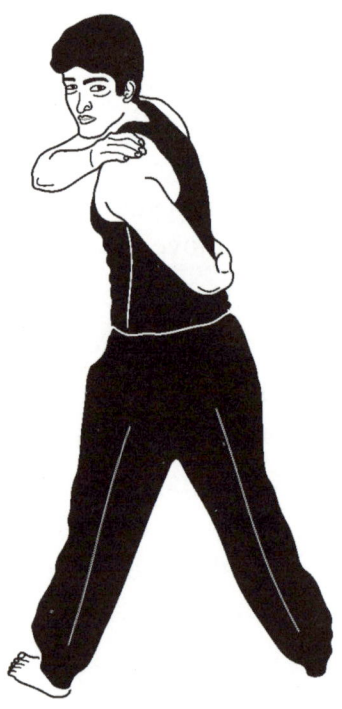

- Stand with legs apart.
- Spread your arms to the sides and take a deep breath.
- Exhaling, turn to your left. Place the right hand on your left shoulder and the left hand on the back of your waist with the palms spread outwards.
- Turn your head and try to look at your heels (over your shoulder).
- Inhaling, return to the centre.
- Exhaling, turn to your right, placing your left hand on your right shoulder and your right hand on the back of your waist and look at your feet.
- Inhaling, centre your body.
- Repeat 4 times.

Triyak Bhujangasana

- Lie down on your stomach.
- Place your hands on both sides near your chest.
- Keep your face down.
- Inhaling, raise your body (the part above your waist) keeping your abdomen firmly on the ground.
- Turn your head to the left to look at your feet over the left shoulder.
- Exhaling, return to the starting position on the ground.
- Practise on the right side.
- Repeat 4 times.

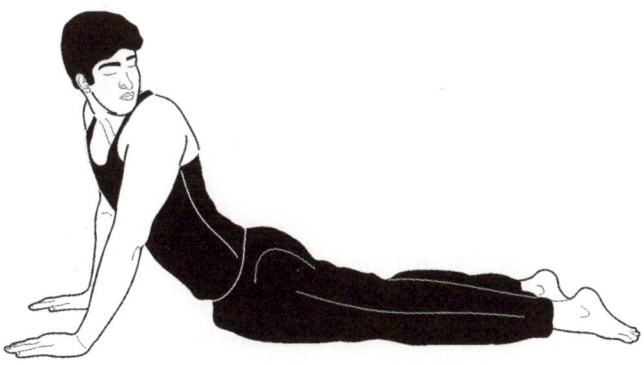

Udarakh

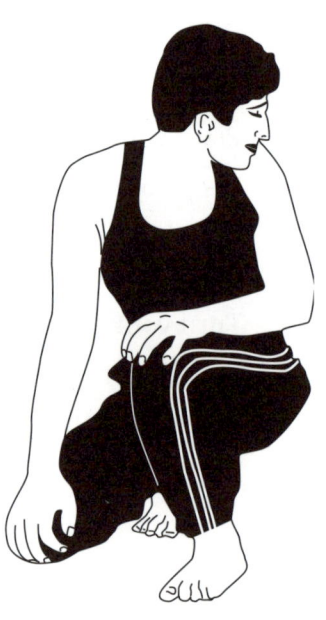

- Squat on the floor with your hands on your knees.
- Raise your heels, and inhaling, turn to your left and put your right knee down on the floor beside the left foot.
- Exhaling, return to the starting position.
- Repeat on the other side to complete one round.
- Practise 4 rounds.
- After performing these five *asana*s, drink two more glasses of water and repeat the process.

The entire cycle is to be carried out three times. After you are done, you can relieve your bowels. If you do not feel the urge to do so, walk around (on your toes, if possible) and do not sit down. After a while, the water will force the intestine to move faster and you will have the urge to evacuate.

Although *Yogasana*s are generally done slowly, *Laghoo Shankha Prakshyalan* needs to be done fast. The sequence of asanas must not be changed, as it is designed to churn the waste from the stomach downwards in a specific sequence.

Laghoo Shankha Prakshyalana can be done every day, but without salt. Salt should be added in the first five to six days and then once a fortnight.

Half an hour after evacuating your bowel, you should do *kunjal*.

KUNJAL

Kunjal, too, is a *satkarma* meant to wash the stomach and remove the acids and bile. At the same time, the movement stimulates the *Manipura Chakra* located on the spine behind the navel. This *chakra* supplies *prana* to the digestive organs speeding up their function.

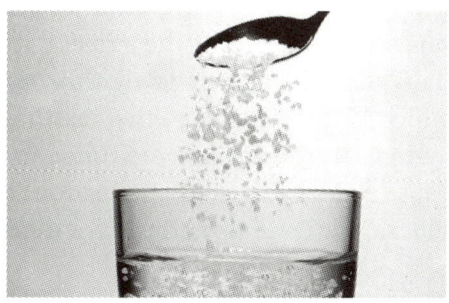

Technique

- Drink three to four glasses of lukewarm saline water quickly as done earlier.
- Bending over a washbasin, insert the first two fingers of your right hand into your mouth and touch or press the throat. The water will gush out. Continue till there is no water left in the stomach. Wait for at least half an hour before eating or drinking anything.

CAUTION: Both Laghoo Shankh Prakshyalan and Kunjal are not meant for people with high blood pressure, heart ailments, hernia and ulcer.

Neti

When we inhale too much dust and other foreign matters, the body tries to trap them by producing more mucus in the respiratory tract. The combined substance can lead to a decreased flow of oxygen and *prana* into the lungs. Furthermore, the crust buries the tiny hair and blood vessels of the nasal passage, which is detrimental to the health of our entire system. Wrong food and infections can also cause excessive mucus production. And too much mucus in the body can create *pranic* blockages. To remove the extra mucus from the nose, *neti* is the most effective means.

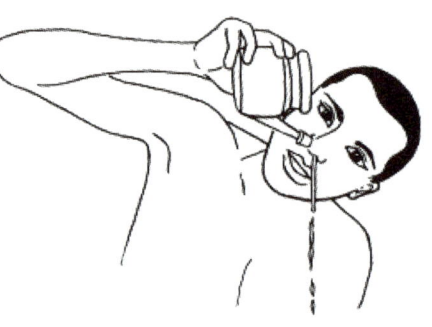

Technique:

- Heat four glasses of water to a luke warm temperature. (The temperature should be slightly more than that of the body.)
- Add approximately one tsp of salt (It should taste as salty as your tear drop.)
- Pour half the water in a neti pot.
- Stand near the washbasin and insert the spout of the pot into your left nostril.
- Start breathing from your mouth.

- Bend forward and tilt your head to the right as you lift the pot. Let the water flow out from your right nostril till the pot is empty.
- Still breathing from your mouth, remove the pot and blow your nose.
- Repeat the procedure for the other nostril as well.
- When it is done, bend forward for half a minute to let the water drain completely. To ensure perfect drainage, you can practise *Shanshankasana* and *Adhvasana* for half a minute each.
- Lastly, practise *Kapalbhati Pranayama* twenty times from the left nostril, twenty times from the right, and twenty times with both nostrils open.

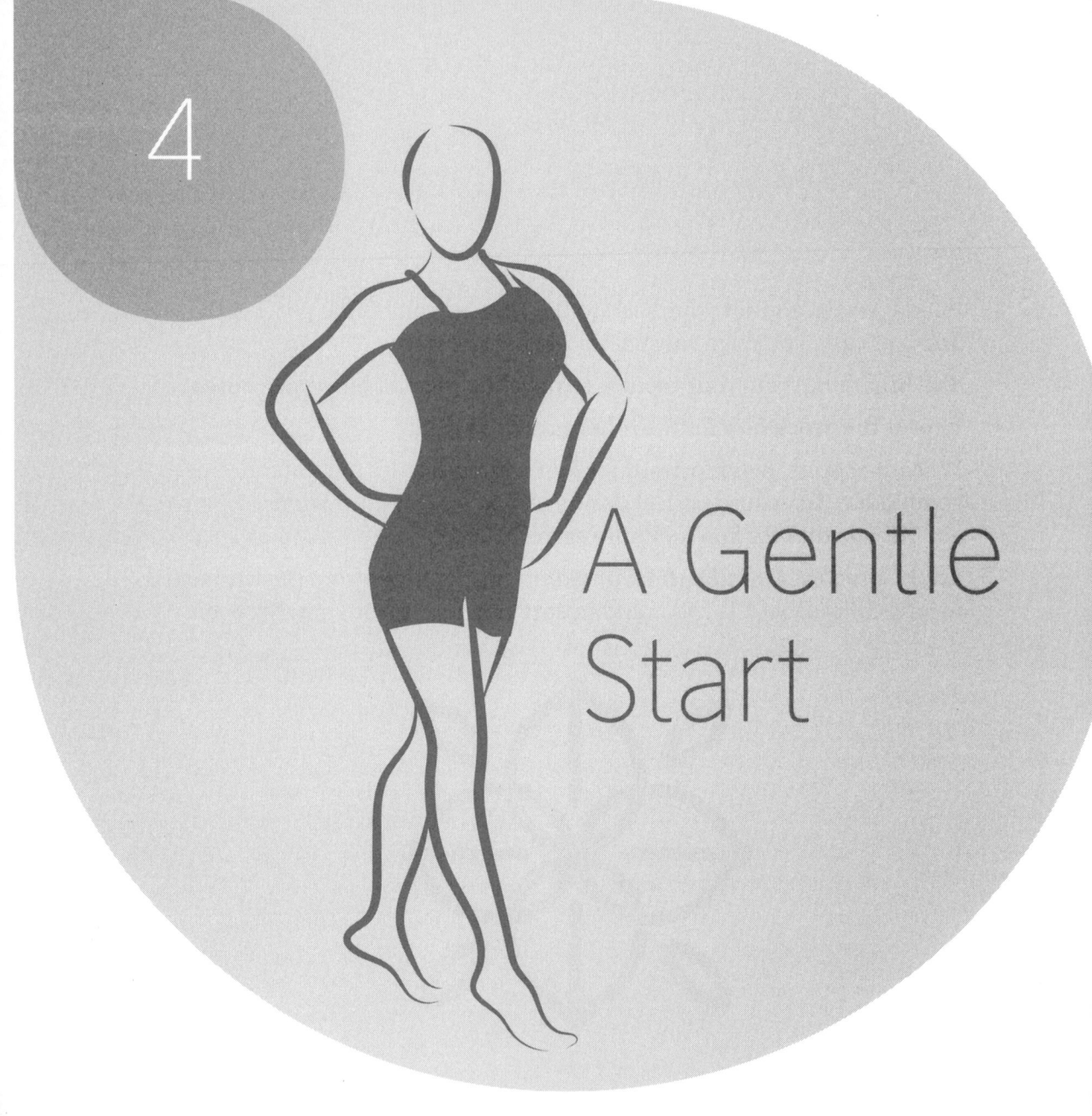

4

A Gentle Start

A Gentle Start

'Use it or lose it' is a famous saying. Very true. Unused muscles gradually become weak and stiff. Unfortunately, in our daily life, we generally do not use many muscles. If these weak hardened muscles are suddenly made to work, they can get damaged. Therefore, before doing the major exercises given in the later chapters, which will put many inactive body parts into action, it is necessary to first make the muscles soft and pliable.

Yoga has a set of simple exercises called *pawanamuktasana,* which works on all the muscles of the body gently in the right way. To be on the safer side, only these practices should be done for the first two to three days, especially if the practitioner has a stiff body or is not too young.

PAWANAMUKTASANA Apart from putting all the muscles into motion in a gentle manner, these exercises squeeze toxins and gases from the tissues. These substances also make the body stiff. The toxins are then pushed into the blood stream, which is then carried to the eliminating organs to be thrown out of the system.

Technique
- Sit down on the floor and stretch your legs in front. Keep your hands on the floor behind your body.

a. Toes bending
- Keeping the feet vertical bend only the toes forward and backwards. The movement should not be too fast or too slow.
- Repeat 10 times.

b. Feet bending
- In the same way, bend the feet forward and backwards from the ankles.
- Repeat 10 times.

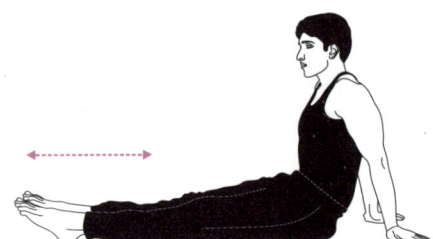

c. Feet rotation
- Move legs apart.
- Rotate both the feet in one direction 10 times and then in the other direction 10 times.

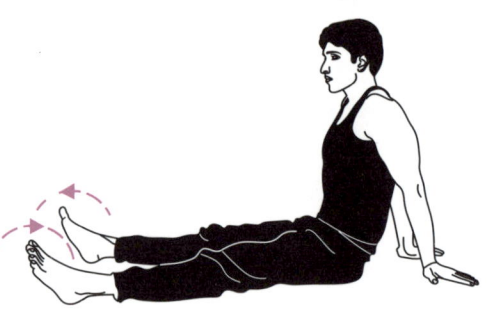

d. Ankle rotation

- Place the right foot on the left thigh; and the right hand on the right knee.
- Holding the right foot with the left hand, rotate it 10 times in one direction, then 10 times in the other direction.
- Repeat with the other leg.

e. Leg bending

- Hold the right thigh with both hands.
- Bend the leg, pulling the knee all the way to the chest and toes pointing upward.
- Straighten the leg with the toes stretched out.
- Repeat 10 times
- Repeat the exercise with the left leg.

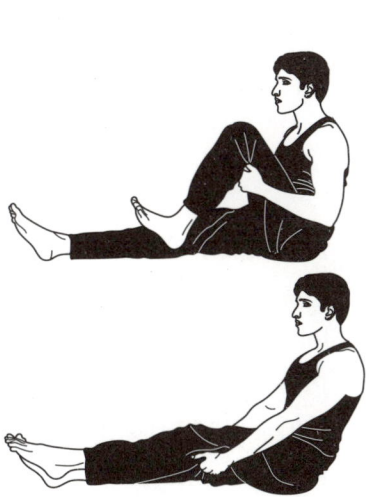

f. Spinal twist

- Move legs wide apart and stretch your arms out.
- Twist your body to the left and touch the left foot with the right hand while the left arm remains undisturbed.
- Return to the starting position.
- Repeat on the other side.
- Repeat 10 times.
- The movement should be continuous.

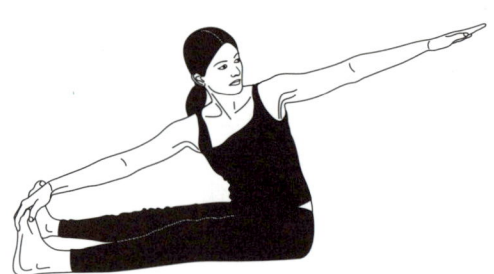

g. Knee pressing

- Keep the right foot on the left thigh.
- Place the right hand on the right knee and the left hand on the left knee.
- Press the right knee down to the floor and then release the pressure.
- Repeat 10 times.
- Repeat the exercise with the left foot.

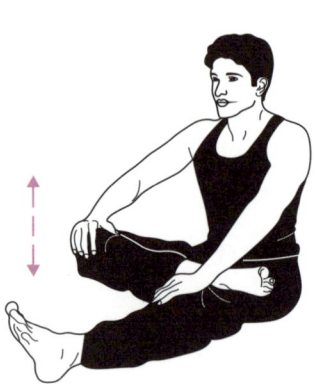

h. Knee rotation

- Keep the right foot on the left thigh close to the body, and hold the foot with your left hand.
- Hold the right knee with your right hand and rotate the knee 10 times in one direction and 10 times in the other direction.
- Straighten the legs and relax.
- Do the same with the left knee.

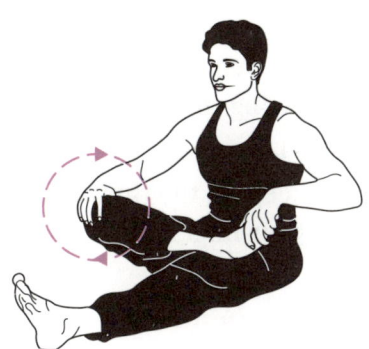

i. Butterfly

- Bend the legs and join the feet facing each other.
- Holding the feet as close to your body as possible, quickly flap the legs up and down a 100 times.
- Straighten the legs and relax.

To do the *asana*s for the upper body, sit with your legs crossed (sukhasna) or keep them extended if you are more comfortable in that position.

Vajrasana also can be assumed if *Sukhasana* is uncomfortable.

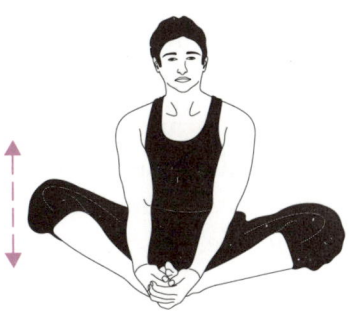

j. Fingers clenching

- Stretch your arms in front with the palms facing the wall and the fingers spread out.
- Clench and flex the fingers 10 times, keeping the thumb in when you clench your fingers.

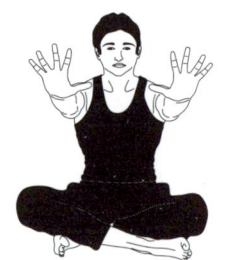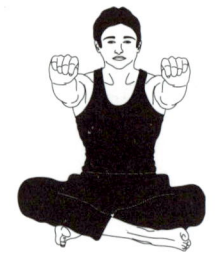

k. Wrist bending

- Stretch the arms out in front with the fingers joined together and palms facing downwards.
- Bend the hands up and down.
- Repeat 10 times.

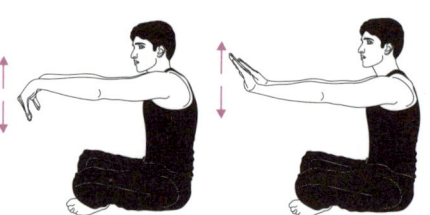

l. Wrist rotation

- Holding the arms in the same position, close the hands into fists with the thumbs inside.
- Rotate the wrists 10 times in one direction and 10 times in the other.

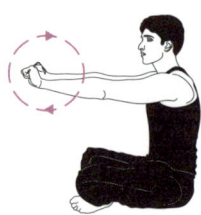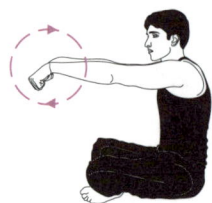

m. Elbow bending

- Holding the arms again in the same extended position and palms facing up, bend them to touch the shoulders with your fingers.
- Straighten them.
- Repeat 10 times.

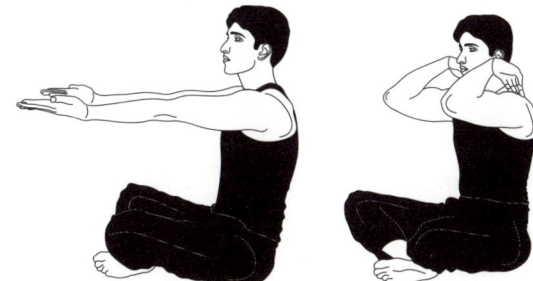

n. Shoulder rotation

- Touch your shoulders with the fingers of the respective hands and rotate your shoulders 10 times in one direction and 10 times in the other.

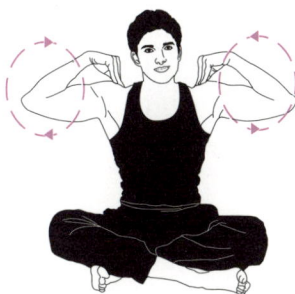

o. Head bending

- Bend the head towards the left shoulder and then towards the right shoulder.
- Repeat 10 times.
- Now bend it forward and backward 10 times.

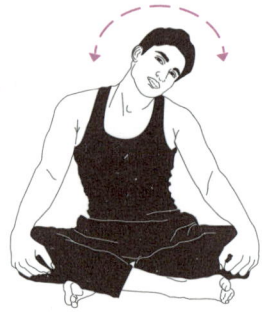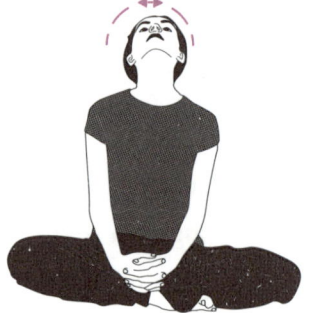

p. Head rotation

- Rotate the head slowly five times in one direction and five times in the other direction.

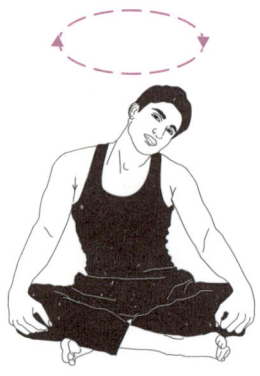

The last two exercises should not be practised by those suffering from cervical spondylitis.

Lie down in *Shavasana* for 10 breaths, counting them backward.

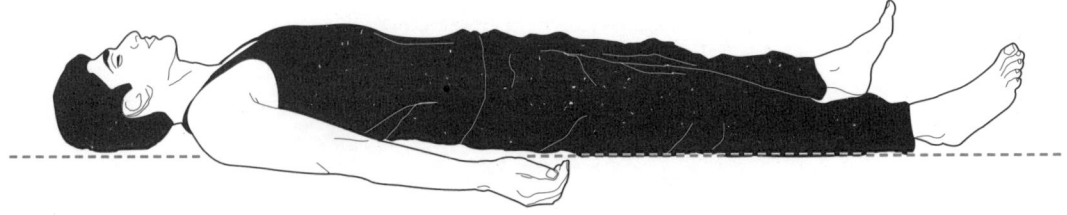

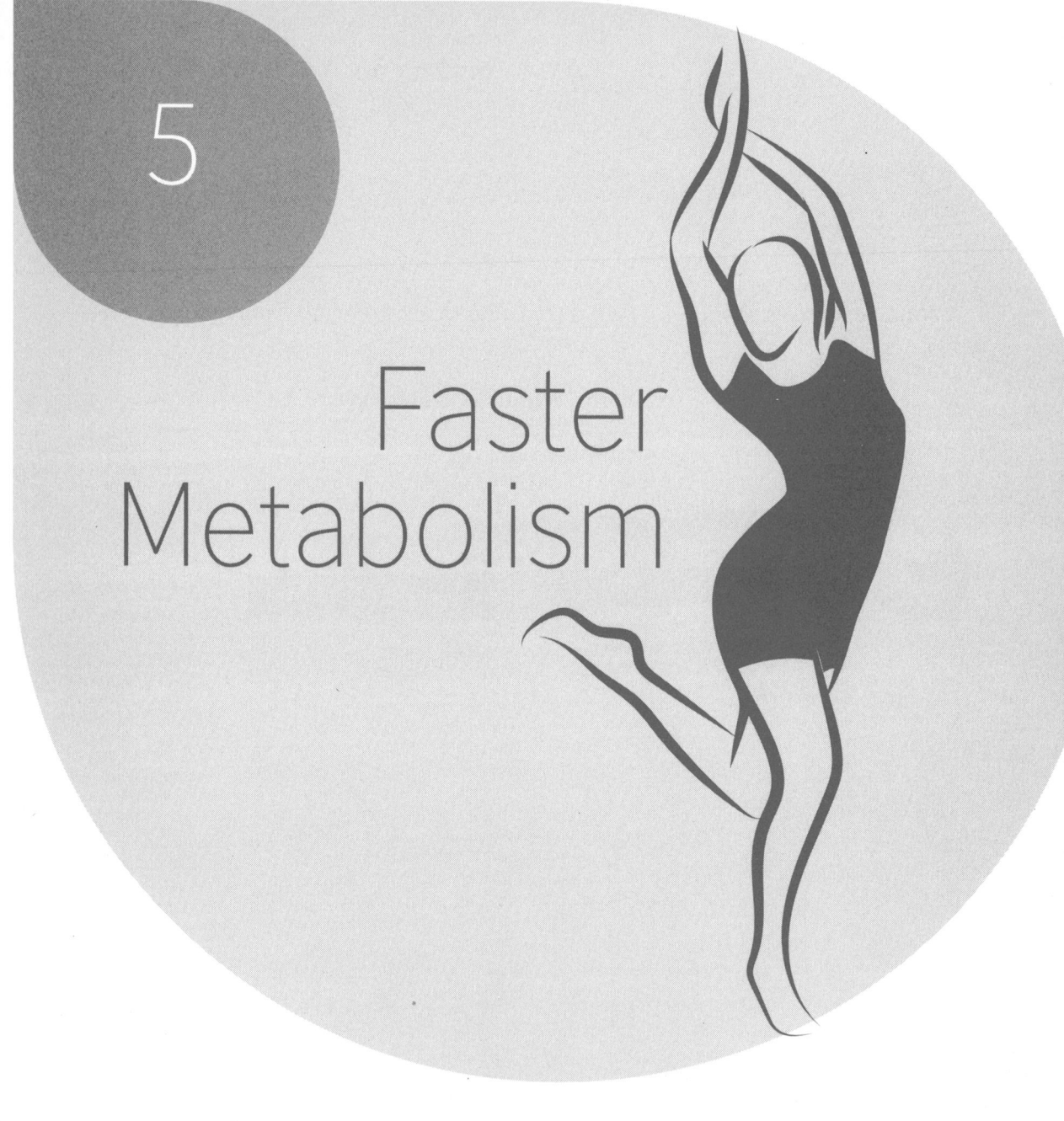

Faster Metabolism

To improve the thyroid health and hasten metabolism, the right *asanas* have to be practised in the right way following all the rules strictly, otherwise one may not get the desired result. Often people treat *asanas* like any other physical exercises which is a mistake. *Asanas* may look like ordinary exercises but are very different in their effects.

Asanas were devised by enlightened masters who had an instinctive knowledge of the human system and the life force. They developed these postures not for the muscles and tissues but mainly to affect the subtle energy system of the body, in specific ways. *Asanas*' main job is to remove blockages from the *nadis* and ensure proper *pranic* flow to a target area. At the same time, they work on the gross body too. With their unique stretching, flexing and twisting, they squeeze out the stagnant toxic blood from the tissues, which is then sent out for elimination. Furthermore, *asanas* are designed to draw extra blood to specific body parts to nourish the weak tissues better. For that purpose, the posture is to be held for a specific duration. Only then the blood can remain around the tissues repairing the damage and strengthening them well. Hence, all major healing *asanas* are static in nature.

Of all the static *asanas*, the inverted ones are most effective for the thyroid, as in such a position, blood naturally flows down to the head and pools around the thyroid. In the subtle level, inverted *asanas* put pressure on the Visuddhi Chakra, which is located at the base of the throat, and stimulate it. Then the chakra is able to supply the necessary amount of *prana* to the thyroid.

SARVANGASANA

This is an inverted *asana* and the main one for the thyroid. This *asana* exerts a great pressure on the gland and activates it properly.

Technique

- Lie down on the floor on your back.
- Placing your hands under your trunk, throw the body up to a vertical position.
- The head and shoulder should remain on the ground with the chin touching the chest.
- Breathe normally. Starting with 5-10 breaths, gradually increase the number of breaths to 60 or more. Then slowly lower your legs and assume *Vipareet Karani Mudra*.
- The effect of *Sarvangasana* is still enhanced if *Ujjayi Pranayama* is practised instead of normal breathing. But this *pranayama* should not be done if the blood pressure is low or if the heartbeat is slow. (See page 49 for *Ujjayi Pranayama*)

CAUTION: Sarvangasana should not be done if you have heart ailments, high blood pressure, vertigo, cervical spondylitis, during pregnancy, enlarged liver, or if your blood is toxic.

Sarvangasana should be preceded by *Dhanurasana*.

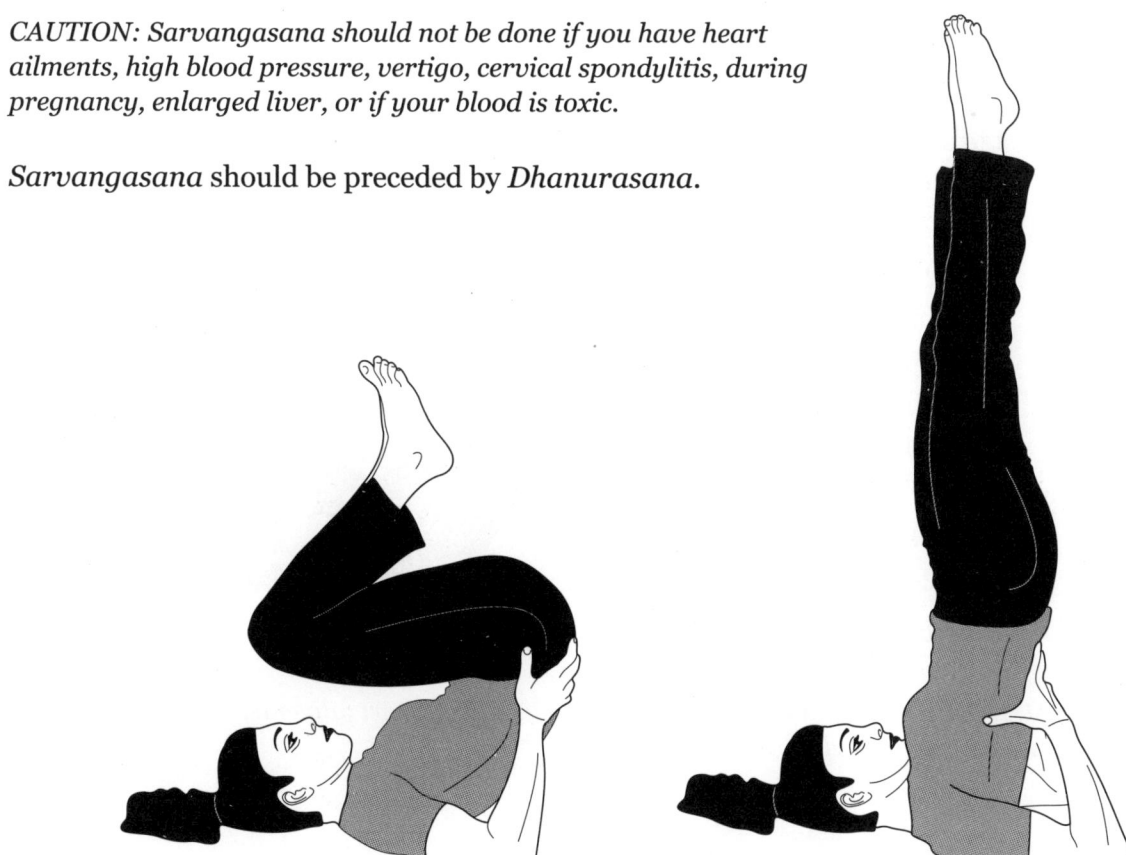

Dhanurasana

Technique

- Lie down on your stomach with legs apart.
- Bend the knees and hold the ankles.
- Inhaling, raise your head and lift the legs up.
- Hold the posture for a comfortable duration.
- Exhale and return to the starting position.
- After 2-3 breaths, repeat.
- Practise three times.

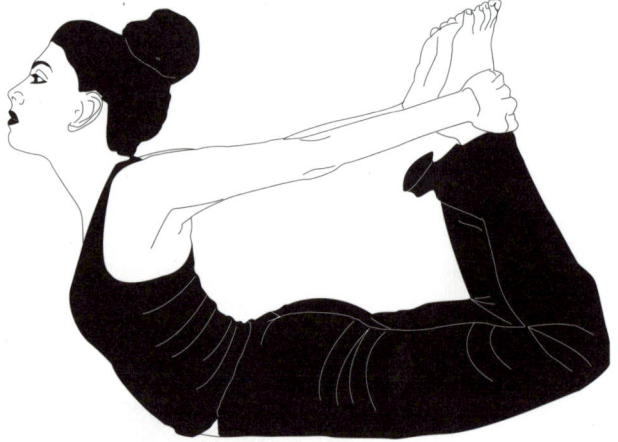

CAUTION: This asana should not be done if you have heart ailments, high blood pressure, stomach ulcer, hernia and colitis.

Vipareet karani mudra

Although this *asana* does not put any pressure on the thyroid, it stimulates certain *nadis* which increases the *pranic* flow to this gland and improves its health.

Technique

- From *Sarvangasana*, lower the hip slightly so that your trunk is held at a sixty degree angle, while the legs remain perpendicular.
- Breathe normally or in *Ujjayi*.
- Starting with 5-10 breaths, gradually increase the number of breaths to 60 or more.

CAUTION: This asana should not be done if you have heart ailments, high blood pressure, vertigo, cervical spondylitis or if the blood is toxic during pregnancy.

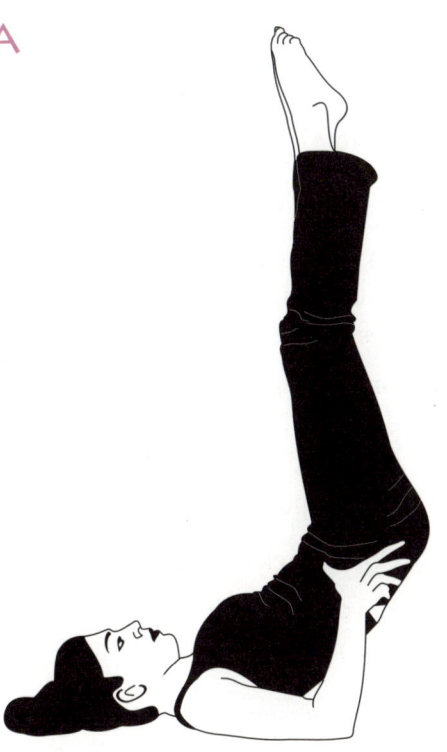

Halasana

Technique

- Maintaining the straight position of the legs, bend them from the hips and place the toes on the ground above your head. Keep your arms on the ground beside your body.
- Breathe normally
- Starting with 5-10 breaths, increase the number of breaths gradually to 30 or more.
- Come back slowly to the starting position.
- Lie down in *Shavasana* for 10-15 or more breaths till your breathing becomes normal.

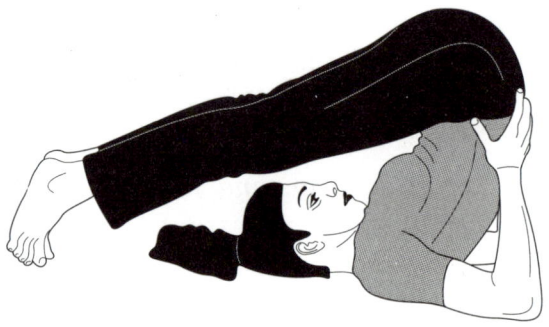

Although Halasana is a static asana, sometimes this asana is added after the two above mentioned asanas and all the three of them are practised in quick succession to make it a dynamic yogic exercise called Druthalasana, which is highly slimming and toning. You can do 5-10 rounds of Druthalasana.

MATSYASANA

Some major *asanas* need to be followed by certain other *asanas* or else there may be adverse consequences. The anti-asana for the three above mentioned *asanas* is *Matsyasana*. The duration of this *asana* has to be the half of the combined duration of all the three *asanas*.

Matsyasana stretches the thyroid, which also draws blood to this gland.

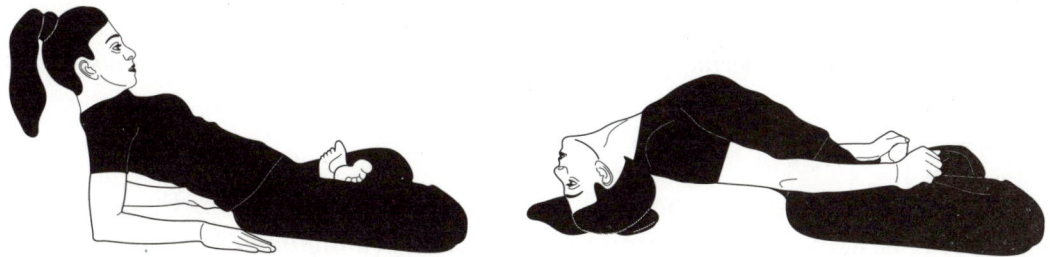

Technique

- Sit in *Padmasana* on a folded blanket or a thick rug.
- Bend backwards.
- Supporting the body with the hands and arching the back, lower the head and place the crown on the ground.

- Hold the toes.
- Breathe normally or in *Ujjayi*.
- Hold the posture for half the combined duration of the three main *asanas*.
- Rise to the starting position and unlock the legs.
- Lie down in *Shavasana* for ten breaths or more till your breathing becomes normal.

CAUTION: This asana should not be done if you have heart ailments, high blood pressure, stomach ulcer, hernia, pregnancy, slipped disc, sciatica or cervical spondylitis.

Matsya Kridasana

Although a resting *asana*, the waist line fat is re-distributed during this posture. It should be done at the end of the *asana* session before *pranayamas*. It can also be done on its own at any other time when the stomach is empty.

Technique

- Lie down on your left side with the left arm extended upwards.
- Bend the right leg and keep the knee close to the chest.
- Bend the right arm and place the elbow on the right leg.
- Bend the left arm to hold the hands.

- Make yourself comfortable by turning your body down.
- Keep the left leg straight.
- Breathe normally for one minute (twenty to twenty-five breaths).
- Repeat on the other side.

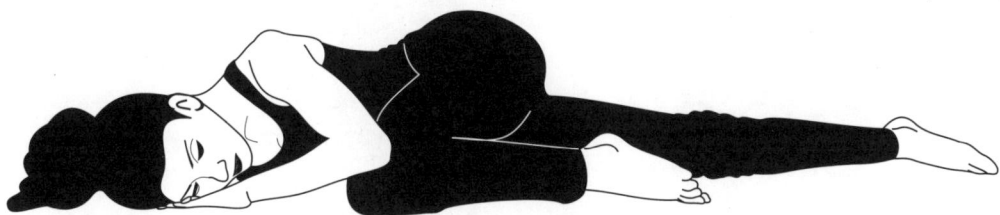

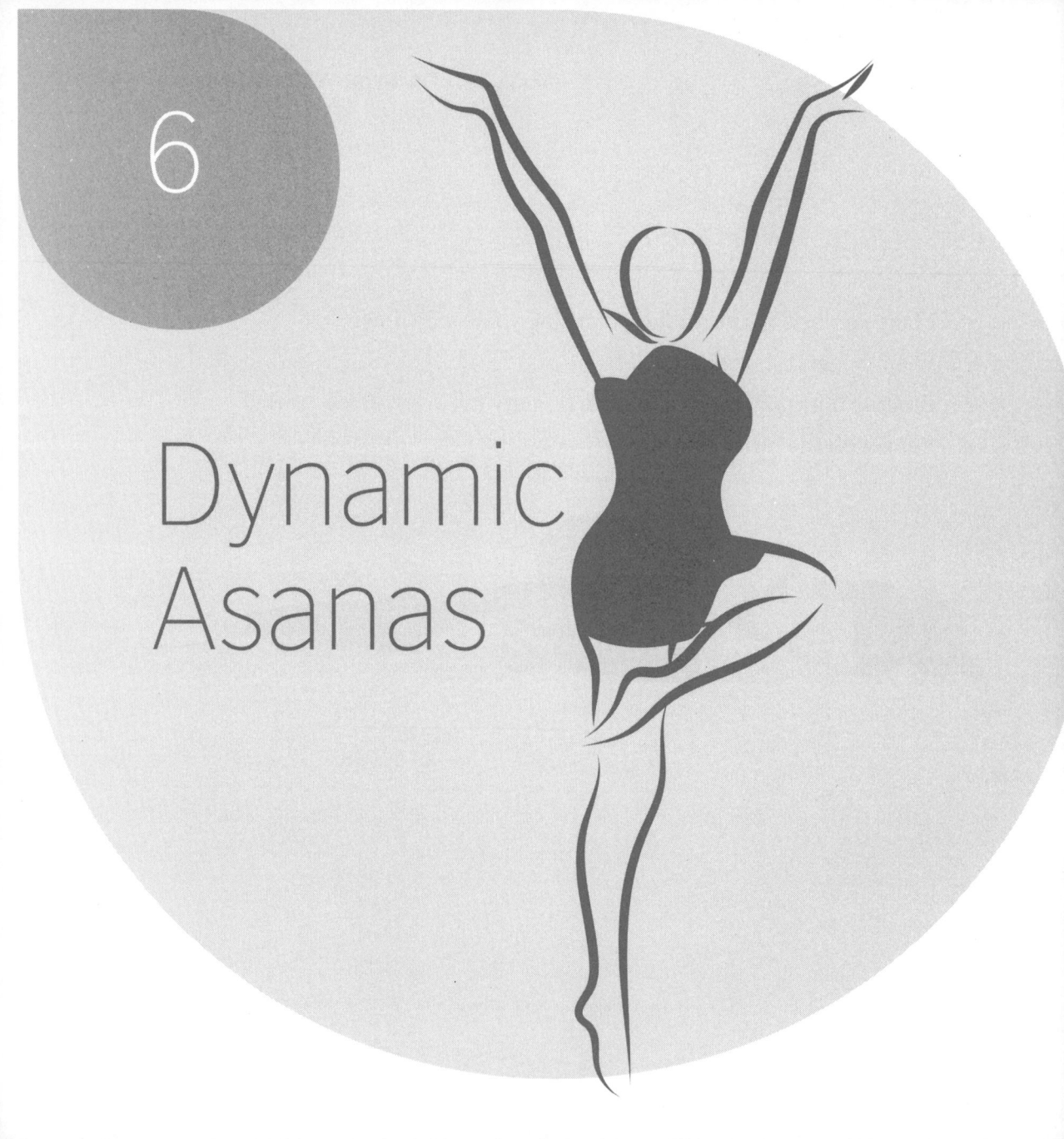

6
Dynamic Asanas

Dynamic Asanas

The *asanas* used to counter obesity are of two kinds—static *asanas* that hold blood around the thyroid to improve its function, and dynamic ones that require more energy resulting in burning of more calories.

Suryanamaskar, which literally meaning 'sun salutation', is the most effective dynamic yogasanas for health and slimming. This exercise is a combination of seven *asanas*, each meant to stretch, flex and exercise a particular body part. Together they cover every inch of the body. As the *asanas* are practised without a break, the movement becomes continuous and at times strenuous. That calls for a supply of high energy, which the body provides by melting the stored fat.

Although most *asanas* are practised less than ten times, *Suryanamaskar* is an exception. One can practise it as many times as one wants—up to 108 rounds. I know of people who practise 108 rounds of this exercise and eat and drink whatever they fancy without putting on any extra weight. My own teacher Swami Swaroopananda Saraswati was doing that when I was in the ashram initially for my treatment.

For most people, it may not be possible or practical to do that many rounds of *Suryanamaskar*. Fifty rounds for men and 25 rounds for women is a good target. But the number should be increased gradually, watching out for a feeling of fatigue. One should feel more energetic after the practice, not drained. If you feel the lack of energy for three consecutive days, reduce the number of rounds.

SURYANAMASKAR

Technique

- 1st step: Stand straight with your feet together and hands folded in a *'namaskar'* (greeting) gesture, in front of your chest.
- 2nd step: Inhaling, lift your arms above your head. Turn your face upwards to stretch the neck, and bend a little backward.
- 3rd step: Exhaling, bend forward and place the hands on the floor (a little in front and outside the feet). You may bend the knees initially, if necessary.
- 4th step: Inhaling, extend the left leg all the way back and bring the hips down while bending the head backward. The right knee should be pointing forward.
- 5th step: Exhaling, lift the bottom up and take the right foot back to join the left one putting the head in between the arms (Do not disturb the position of the hands henceforth)
- 6th step: Holding out the breath, lower your body to rest on the ground, but make sure that the bottom is held up and the hands are beside the chest.

- 7th step: Drop the pelvic to the floor, and inhaling, lift your head, then the chest and then the stomach all the way up to straighten the arms. Turn the head back to stretch the neck well.
- 8th step: Exhaling, return to the fifth position.
- 9th step: Inhaling, return to the fourth position.
- 10th step: Exhaling, return to the third position.
- 11th step: Inhaling, return to the second position.
- 12th step: Exhaling, return to the first position.
- Repeat on the other side, i.e., extend the right leg back.
- These two cycles form one round.
- Starting with one round, gradually increase the number of rounds.

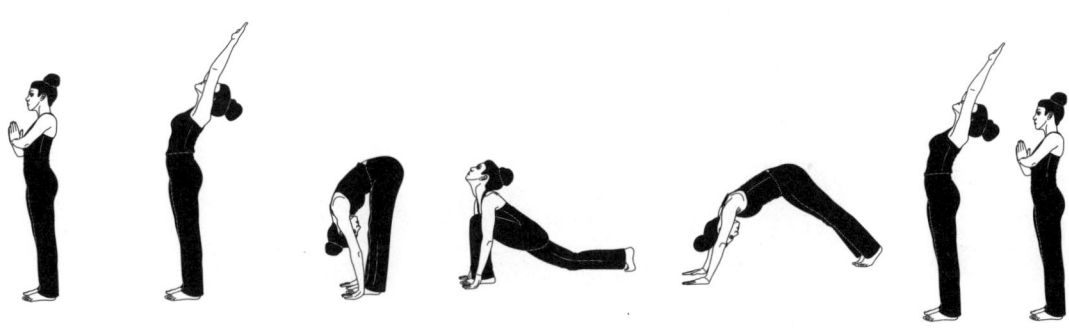

After *Suryanamaskar*, it is necessary to lie down in *Shavasana* till the breathing becomes normal. Generally, 10 breaths per one round is needed.

CAUTION: Suryanamaskar should not be done if you have heart ailments, high blood pressure, hernia, stomach ulcer or any kind of back problem.

SHAVASANA

In this *asana*, the tension is released from all the muscles of the body.

Technique

- Lie down on your back, with the legs around 18 inches apart.
- Move your hands a little away from the body with the palms facing up.
- Close your eyes.
- Breathe naturally.
- Count your breaths backwards.

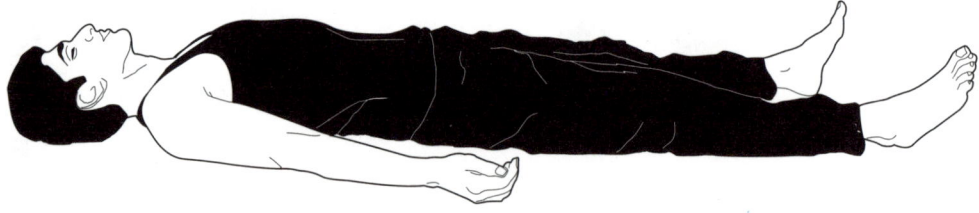

Other dynamic asanas

Padahastasana

Technique

- Stand straight with feet joined.
- Inhaling, raise your hands and stretch your body well, bending a little backward.
- Exhaling, bend forward and touch your feet.
- Inhaling, return to the starting position.
- Repeat 10-15 or even 20 times.

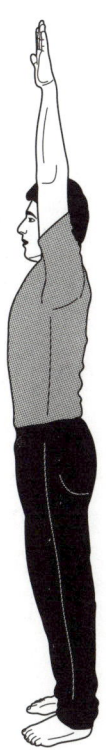
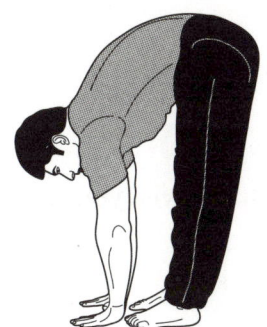

Meru pristasana 1

Technique

- Stand straight with legs apart.
- Touch your shoulders with your fingers.
- Exhaling, bend to your left side.
- Inhaling, return to the standing position.
- Repeat 10-15 times.
- Repeat the same on the right side.

Meru pristasana 2

Technique

- Assume the same posture like as previous *asana*.
- Take a deep breath.
- Holding your breath in, twist your trunk to the left.
- Exhaling, bend forward.

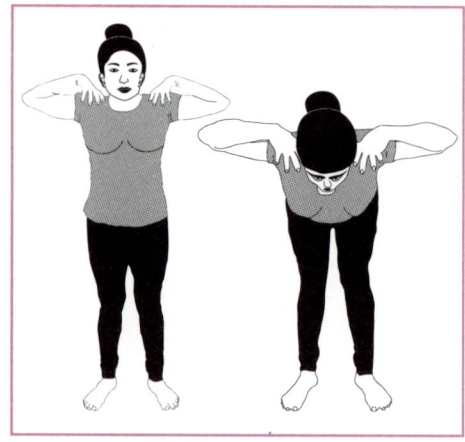

- Inhaling, straighten up.
- Holding the breath in twist to the right.
- Exhaling, bend forward.
- Repeat 10-15 times.

SWINGING KATICHAKRASANA
Technique
- Stand straight with legs apart .
- Extend your arms in front.
- Inhale.
- Exhaling, swing to the left.
- Inhaling, return.
- Exhaling, swing to the right side and repeat the process 10-15 times.
- Maintain the position of the arms throughout the practice.

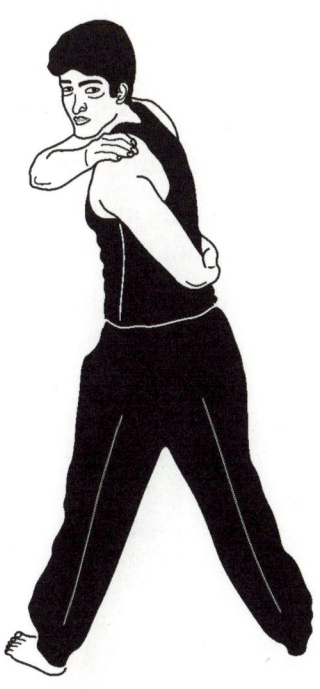

Trikonasana

All the variations of Trikonasana are for slimming and, at the same time, they strengthen the nervous system.

Technique

Trikonasana-1

- Stand with your feet apart and arms extended to the sides.
- Exhaling and bending the left knee, bend your body to the left and touch the left foot with your left hand while turning the face up to look at the ceiling.
- Bring the right arm down to a horizontal position.

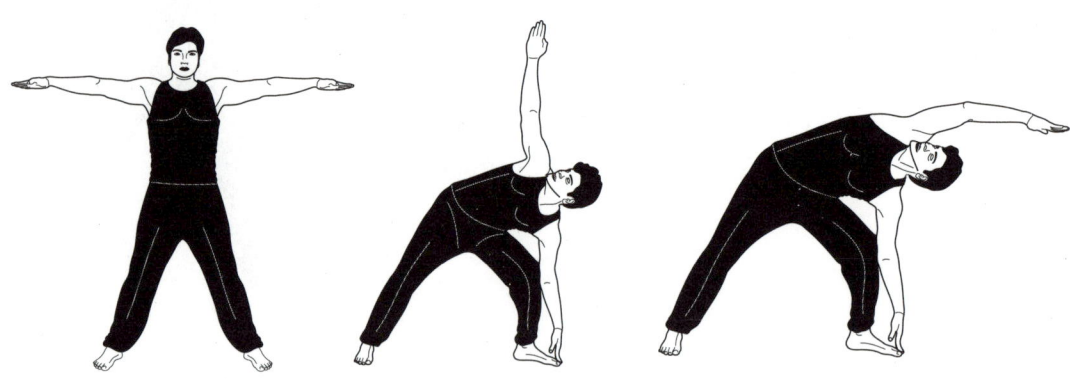

- Inhaling, return to the starting position and repeat on the other side to complete a round.
- Practise 10-15 rounds.

Trikon-2

- Stand with your feet apart and hands clasped behind.
- Take a deep breath.
- Bend the left knee, and exhaling, bend forward to touch the left knee with your nose.
- Inhaling, straighten up.
- Practise on the right side to complete a round.
- Repeat 10-15 times.

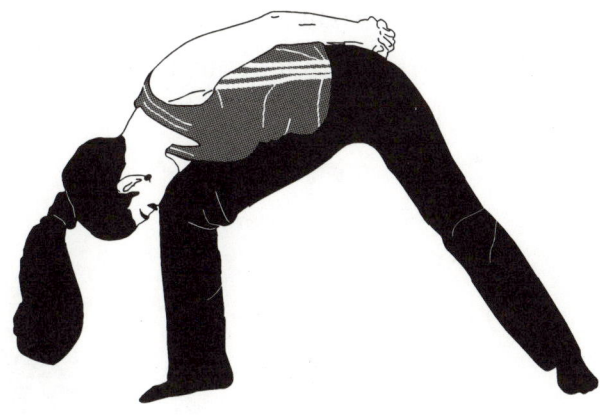

Trikon-3

- Stand with your feet apart and arms extended on the sides.
- Exhaling, bend forward.
- Holding your breath in, twist the trunk and touch the left foot with the right hand while turning the head back over the left shoulder; and again twisting to the other side, touch the right foot with the left hand while turning the head over the right shoulder; then return to the bent posture.
- Inhaling, return to the starting upright position.
- Repeat 10-15 times.

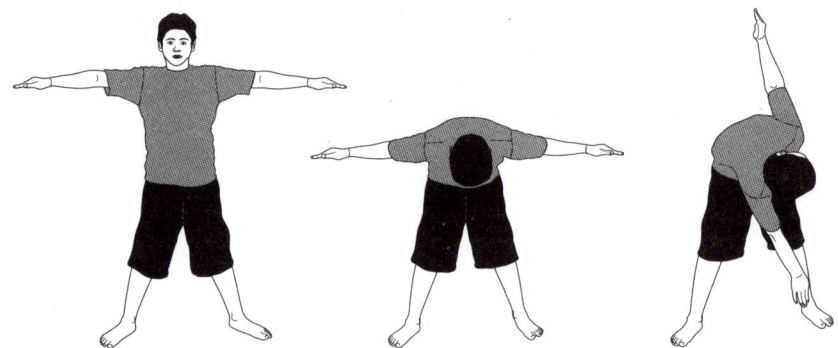

There are very effective dynamic asanas for each part of the body. If you have any particular area that has a tendency to hold on to fat, then you should add the relevant spot reduction asanas. (See my book 'Yoga to preserve Youth & Beauty'.)

Yoga and Diet for Weight Loss

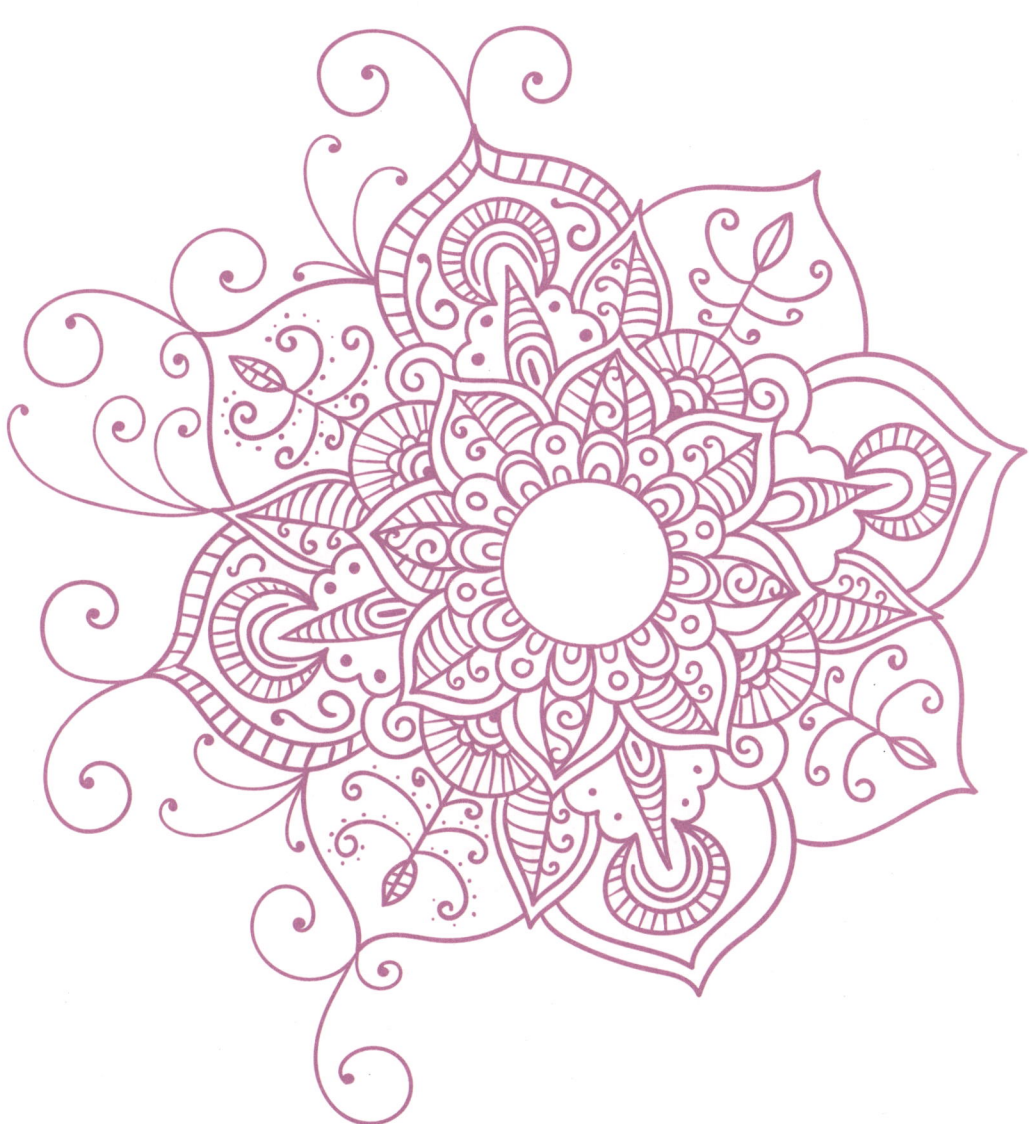

7

Prana Enhancer

Prana Enhancer

Prana the bio current gets used up by the body cells and needs to be replenished from time to time. Although this energy enters the body automatically, *pranayamas* ensure a greater volume. Also, they carry the *prana* to the right places in the body.

There are many *pranayamas*, each with specific effects on the system. Some are heating, some are cooling, some lower blood-pressure and some increase it. Therefore, they should be chosen carefully according to the body's condition and needs. If a hypertensive person does a pranayam that is meant to elevate the blood pressure, he or she can be in trouble.

Nadisodhana Pranayama is the most common and essential *pranayama*, and it suits all types. As the name suggests, this *pranayama* is meant to purify the 'nadis' or energy channels.

A session of *asanas* must be followed by *pranayamas*, beginning with *Nadisodhan Pranayama*.

All *pranayama* should be practised in a meditative pose such as *Padmasana*, *Siddhasana*, *Vajrasana* or the simple *Sukhasana*.

Padmasana

Technique

- Sit with legs crossed
- The right foot should be on the left thigh and the left foot should be on the right thigh
- Maintain a straight posture

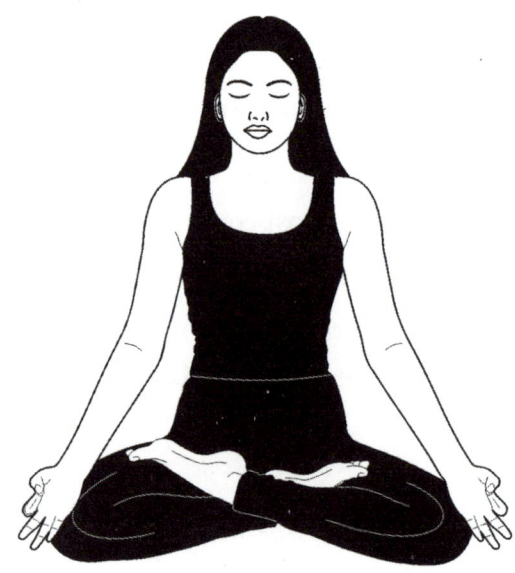

SIDDHASANA

Technique

- Sit with your legs extended in front.
- Bend the right leg and keep the heel pressing against the perineum.
- Bend the left leg and keep the heel pressed against your pubic bone and insert the toes in to the fold of the right leg.
- Pull the toes of the right leg up in between the thigh and calf of the left leg.

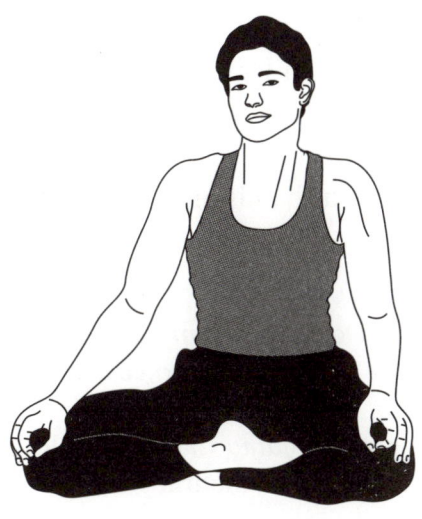

SUKHASANA

- Sit down and simply cross your legs.

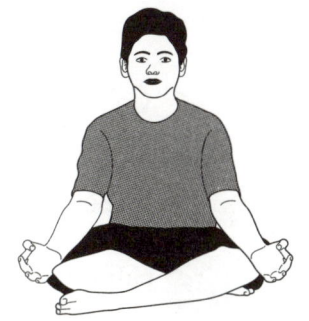

Vajrasana

- Sit with your legs folded underneath—the toes should touch each other but not overlap.
- Place your hands on the thighs.
- Breathe normally.

CAUTION: Do not perform these asanas if you have a knee injury and/or knee arthritis.

During *pranayama*, hands should be held in chin mudra or gyana mudra.

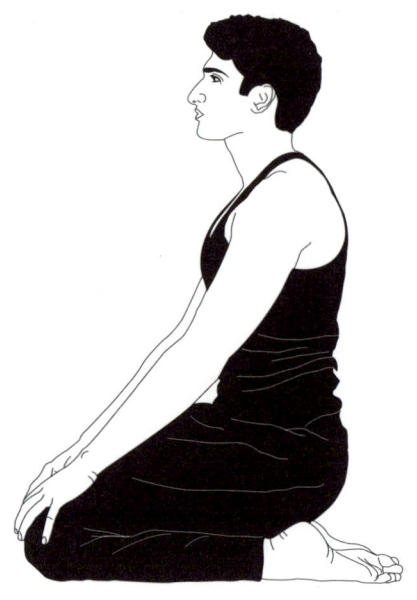

Chin Mudra

Technique

Bend the index fingers of your hands and let the tips touch the base of the thumbs. Place the hands on your knees with the palms facing up.

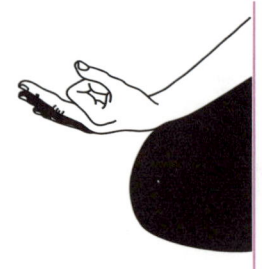

Gyana Mudra

Technique

Same as the previous one, but here the palms face down.

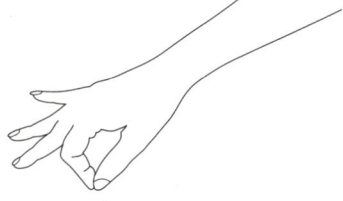

Nadisodhana Pranayama

Technique

First Stage: *(To be practised for a week, and then replaced by the second stage.)*
- Sit in a meditative pose. Keep the left hand on the left knee in chin mudra.
- Place the index and middle finger of the right hand in the space between the eyebrows.
- Close the right nostril with your thumb and breathe normally 10 times from the left nostril.
- Then closing the left nostril with the ring finger, breathe from the right nostril 10 times.

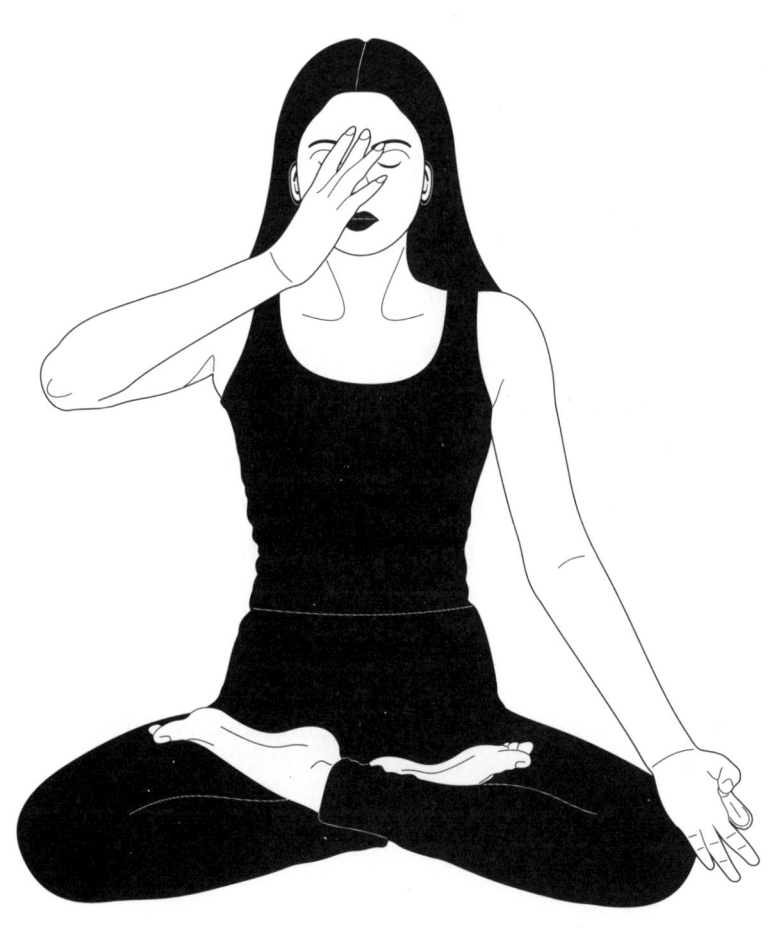

Second Stage: *(To be practised for a week and then replaced by the third stage.)*
- Breathe in from the left nostril. Then closing the left nostril with the ring finger, breathe out from the right nostril.
- Repeat 10 times.
- Practise with the other nostril in the same way.

Third stage: *(To be replaced by the fourth stage after a week.)*
- Assume the same *pranayama* posture.
- Breathe in from the left nostril and breathe out from the right nostril, then breathe in from the right nostril and breathe out from the left nostril.
- Repeat 10 times.

CAUTION: From the third stage onwards, this pranayama is not meant for people with heart ailments and high blood pressure.

Fourth stage: Though there are many more advanced stages, this stage will suffice for slimming.
- Assume the same *pranayama* posture.
- Breathing is similar to the third stage but after inhalation, close both nostrils and hold the breath, maintaining the ratio of 1:1:1—he duration of inhalation, retention and exhalation should be the same.

- To count both the ratios and the number of rounds, it is convenient to do it in the following manner:
  - In the first round, mentally repeat 'one' seven times or whatever number you take to complete your inhalation. Then again repeat 'one' the same number of times while you hold your breath, and again count 'one' the same number of times with exhalation.
  - In the second round, instead of 'one' repeat 'two'.
  - Continue till you finish 'ten'.

Ujjayi pranayama

This is very effective to improve thyroid function. The glottis is contracted to do this *pranayama* which pressurizes the thyroid gland and stimulates it.

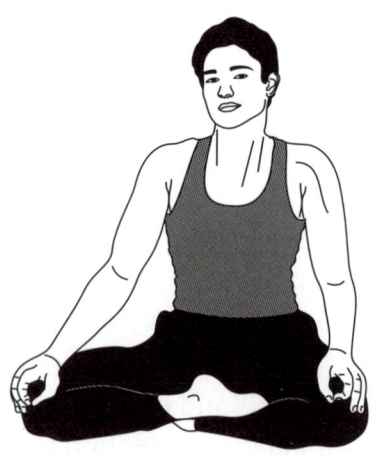

Technique

- Sit in a meditative pose.
- Fold your tongue and close the mouth.
- Breathe from the nose and feel the breath in the throat by constricting the throat area a little.

- The breath should make a hissing sound.
- Adjust the contraction, so that you alone should be able to hear the sound.
- Practise 27 rounds.

CAUTION: This pranayama should not be done if you have low blood-pressure or slow heart beat

Kapalabhati pranayama

This is a vigorous *pranayama,* which accelerates the metabolism of the body and tightens the abdominal muscles.

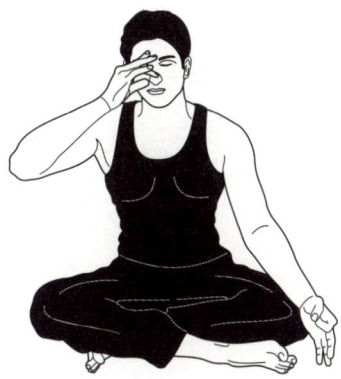

Technique
- Assume the same pose as *Nadisodhan Pranayama.*
- Closing the right nostril with the thumb, breathe vigorously 20 times from the left nostril; then closing the left nostril, breathe 20 times through the right.
- Practise 3 rounds.

CAUTION: This pranayama should not be done if you have heart ailments, high blood pressure, vertigo, epilepsy, stomach ulcer or hernia.

8
Sleep to Succeed

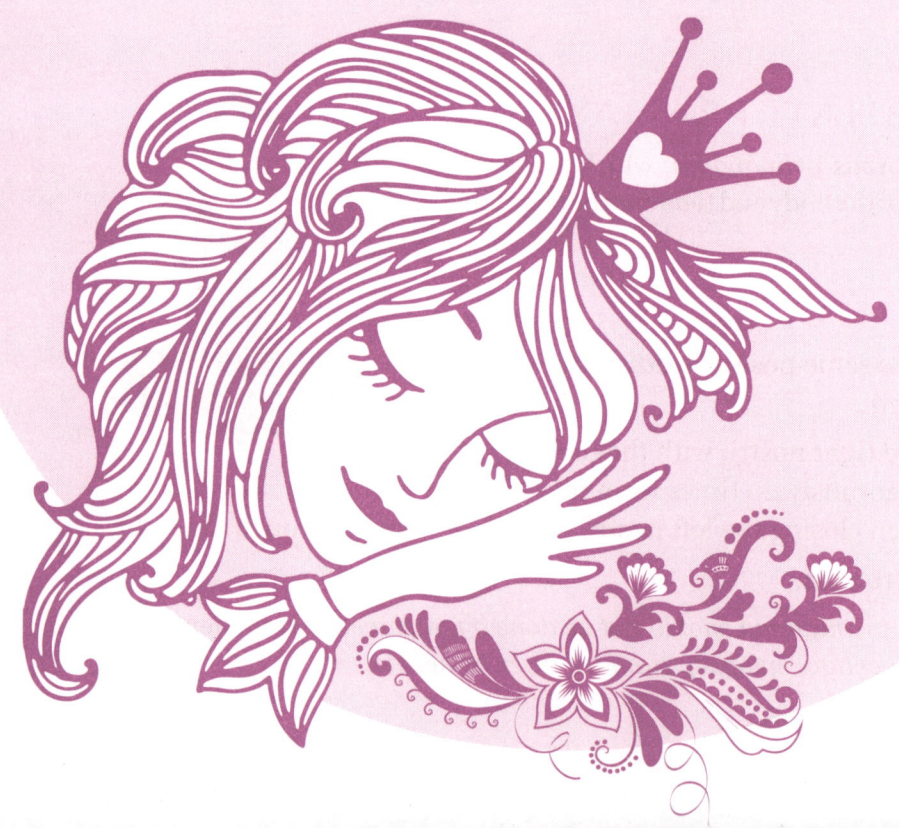

Sleep to Succeed

It is common knowledge that sound sleep is essential for good health. It is only during sleep that the worn out body tissues are repaired and revived. No gland or organ in the body can function properly unless we sleep well. Deeper the sleep, better is the tissue rejuvenation.

Unfortunately in today's world, natural sound sleep is extremely rare. People lead a highly stressful life and carry their stress to bed. The brain remains active thinking and analysing the day's problems. When the mind is thus not relaxed, the body cannot let go of its tension. With a tense body and mind, restful sleep is not possible. Even if one manages to fall asleep in that condition, the sleep generally is not of high quality. The person keeps tossing and turning all through the night and may wake up a few times during that period. Obviously, the body parts do not get a good chance to rejuvenate themselves well. In such a condition, one starts the day with less efficient glands and organs. If it happens for a short period, the body can tolerate it. But trouble starts when it is repeated every night. In the long run, such poor sleep leads to poor health as well as slower metabolism. Also, researchers of the University of Chicago have found that sleep deprived people cannot resist high-calorie snacks such as cookies, candies, chips etc., resulting in weight gain.

Often people turn to sleep medication which is of little value, because many restorative phases are bypassed in medicated sleep. Secondly, drugs are chemicals, and chemicals can interfere with the functioning of the system including that of the thyroid.

Apart from poor sleep, stress itself is bad for the thyroid function as well. The thyroid, situated at the base of our neck is designed to secrete certain hormones, including thyroxin, which controls our metabolism. The amount of thyroxin this gland is to secrete is determined by the pituitary—the master gland. The pituitary gets its instructions from a part of the brain called hypothalamus, and it is this body part that is directly connected with the mind. When the mind is stressed and preoccupied with an external problem, the hypothalamus too gets tense and its judgements can become faulty. Consequently, its erratic orders are relayed to the body via the pituitary and the functions of all the glands and organs can go haywire. That can lead to various problems, including a malfunctioning thyroid.

One cannot avoid stress in this world. It is inevitable in life, as it comes from far too many sources such as career, health, education, relationships, crime, natural calamities, traffic jams, quarrelsome neighbors, noisy children, loud music, inefficient and insincere staff and many more. We can only counter the harmful effects of it, and that can be achieved through certain techniques.

Yoganidra is a very effective de-stressor that was developed by the great guru Paramahamsa Swami Satyananda Saraswati from a tantric ritual, where systematically touching the body parts leads to a completely relaxed state. In *Yoganidra*, one does not need to touch anywhere in the body but just visualize it. By the end of the practice, the entire body is completely relaxed. This practice is so powerful that half an hour of it is seen to have the same effect on the body as two hours of natural deep sleep. Furthermore, one is generally lulled to sleep after *Yoganidra*. The quality of that sleep is very high, which facilitates optimum tissue rejuvenation. Therefore, every weight watcher should sleep with *Yoganidra* for the best health of the thyroid. Insomniacs can do it twice a day because even if they do not sleep for the recommended eight hours a day, their body will still get the rest it needs and does not suffer the effect of sleep deprivation.

Another advantage of *Yoganidra* is that it is an excellent medium to reach the subconscious, and with this mind's help, one can get anything. Attaining a perfect body is nothing for this mind. It is said that through the subconscious, one can even move a mountain. Hence, apart from working on the body, it is essential to work on the mind and make it accept your wish to get what you want from your body.

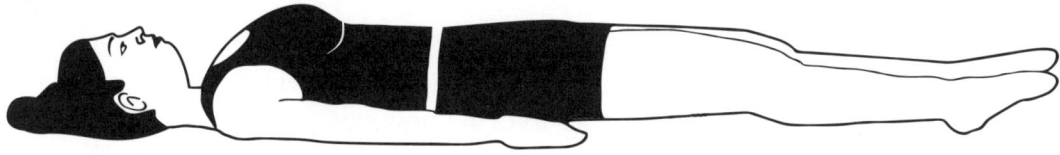

The subconscious mind surfaces and becomes receptive only when the physical body is completely relaxed and the conscious mind is inactive. Such a state is indicated by the alpha brain waves. The brain generally generates the fast beta waves when we are awake and our conscious mind is busy flitting from thought to thought. But during sleep and, very briefly, just before and after sleep when the mind is not active, slow alpha waves are emitted. But during *Yoganidra*, these wave are produced abundantly even when the person is awake indicating the inaction of the conscious mind. A resolve made in that state makes a strong impression on the subconscious which almost always bears fruit.

The resolve must be framed carefully. The sentence should be short and clear and should have a positive note with no negative words in it. A lady who was very fond of cakes and pastries made a mistake of using a negative word in her resolve. She said, 'I will *not* eat any fattening food.' She did not. But every time she saw anything she was tempted to eat, her stomach would start hurting. She could not understand the reason and had to endure the pain till she casually mentioned it to me. I taught her the way to get out of it. But it took her a long time to rectify that error.

Yoganidra is a simple and pleasant practice where one does not need to do anything physically, but just listen to the voice and follow the instructions in the mind. Traditionally, only a live voice was used, but now a days, it is being recorded for convenience and commercial use. You can even record it in your own voice. Choose a pitch that you find most soothing.

Although *Yoganidra* can be done anytime and more than once a day, practising it at bedtime is essential. That way, not only the accumulated tension of the day is removed, but the sleep that follows is the most rejuvenating. Consequently, one gets up feeling fresh and energetic the next morning and finds it easier to do more rounds of the dynamic *Suryanamaskar*. *Yoganidra* should be practised in semi darkness for enhanced effect as the nerves automatically relax in such condition.

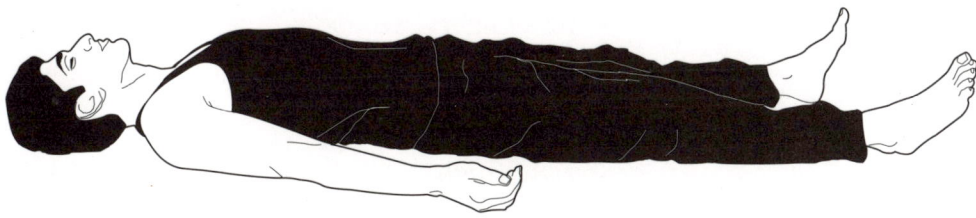

Technique

- Lie down in *Shavasana*.
- Close your eyes gently and relax the body.
- Adjust your body to a very comfortable position.
- Take a deep breath.
- As you exhale, say 'R-e-l-a-x-' in your mind and let the tension leave your body.

- Every time you exhale, say 'R- e- l- a- x-' mentally and try to relax a little more.
- Practise at least 10-15 breaths in this way.
- Now make a resolve and repeat it firmly three times in your mind.
- Then move your mind over the body and visualize the body parts in the following sequence:

Right hand thumb	>	first finger	>	second finger
third finger	>	fourth finger	>	palm
wrist	>	elbow	>	shoulder
right hip	>	right thigh	>	knee
calf	>	ankle	>	heel
sole	>	big toe	>	second toe
third toe	>	fourth toe	>	fifth toe

Repeat with the left side of your body starting with the left hand thumb.

Then go to your back and visualize the following parts:

| Right shoulder | > | left shoulder | > | right side of the back |
| left side | > | right heel | > | left heel |

Then move your mind over the front of your body in the following sequence:

Top of the head	>	forehead	>	right eyebrow
left eyebrow	>	right eye	>	left eye
right ear	>	left ear	>	right cheek
left cheek	>	right nostril	>	left nostril
upper lip	>	lower lip	>	chin
chest	>	abdomen		

Repeat the entire process two to three times more for complete relaxation. Then repeat your resolution three times again, and end the practice.

Recorded Yoganidra has more elements than just the body visualization for healing purposes.

9
Via the Mind

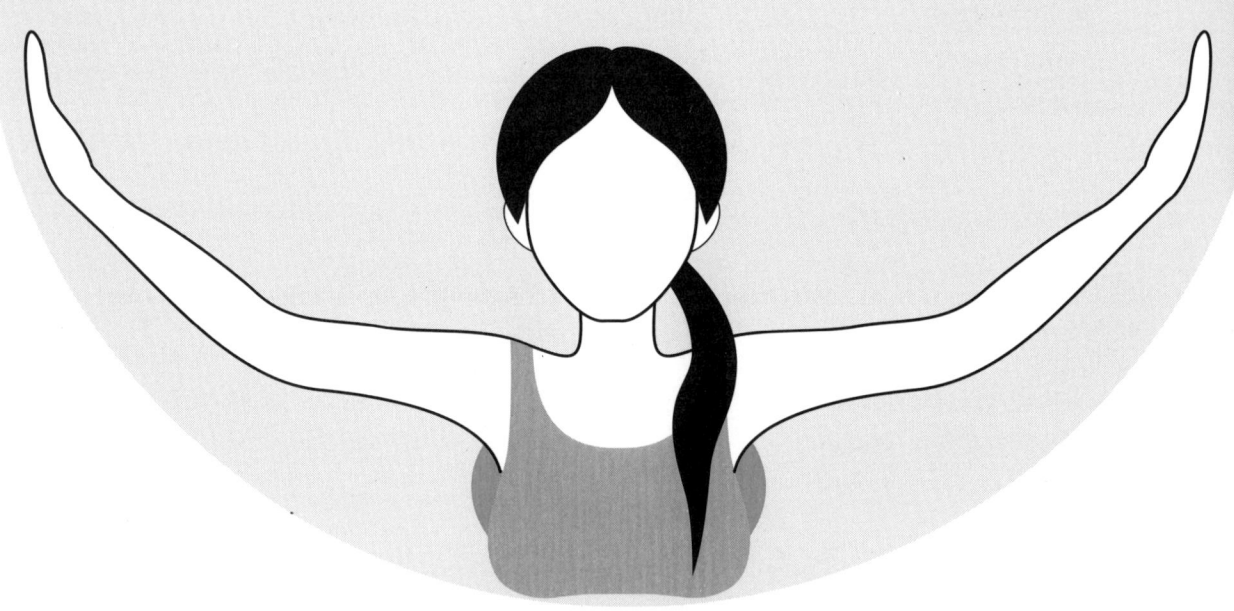

Via the Mind

As has already been mentioned, the power of the subconscious is unlimited. But it goes both ways. If this mind can be turned into a faithful servant who can get you whatever you want, it can also become your stubborn master. It can pass any order and you will have to follow it. If it decides that you should be obese, it can make all your efforts to be otherwise futile. It will slow down your metabolism, make you crave all the high-calorie unhealthy food, and will weaken your desire to do any physical exercises. Even reducing your food to the barest minimum will not bear any result, as the more you decrease your food, the more sluggish your thyroid will become. There is no winning an adverse thinking subconscious.

The subconscious mind's decisions are not arbitrary. Those are based on our own thoughts and inner beliefs. And our belief system is built on our past experiences. Whatever we infer from incidents early in life remains in our inner mind and provides the database for the subconscious calculations. For example, there is a woman who as a child had been quite traumatized seeing somebody with smallpox. The image kept coming to her mind; she just could not get rid of it. After some time, every time she saw a pockmarked person, she would get severe rashes on her face. Perhaps her subconscious mind thought that that was what the girl wanted as she was thinking of the picture so much. The fear of getting the rash made it still worse, as with time, the severity of the problem increased causing still more stress. That led to many other stress related ailments such as high blood pressure, diabetes and indigestion.

It is not just childhood traumas that cause adverse subconscious decisions. In adult life too, stress coming from serious ailments, lack of love, divorce, death and turbulent relationships can influence the subconscious mind to take negative steps.

Fortunately, the subconscious mind can be made to change its way of thinking. For that, first the offending cause that lies buried in the deepest mind has to be rooted out. Although *Yoganidra* can remove the stress of daily life, it is not so effective in dealing with the emotional stress and negative beliefs. Meditation is the only way to achieve that.

Although to an ordinary person *Yoganidra* and meditation seem the same. However, there is a difference between them. It can be seen in the brain wave pattern generated during each practice. During *Yoganidra,* they are mostly alpha, while in meditation, they are still the slower theta and even the slowest delta, which indicates the involvement of a still deeper level of the mind, i.e., the unconscious where the past impressions are stored.

There are innumerable kinds of meditations in the world. Although they all are effective in de-stressing the deeper mind, one needs to choose a practice according to the nature of the stress for quick and satisfactory results. For example, if the stress is acquired from a childhood shock or trauma, a cathartic meditation such as *antarmouna* is most suitable; and if it is due to a deep tragedy, a music meditation is the best answer, as music is known to soothe the mind and the frayed nerves faster.

It is best to consult an expert to select the right meditative practice for yourself. It will save you the time and dilemma. But in case of the absence of such a person, you can do a mantra meditation. This type of meditation is safe, easy and effective. For obesity, repeating the mantras of the 'chakras' or energy centres that control the thyroid and the digestive system, respectively, should be used. Apart from removing the stress from the mind, these mantras will activate the concerned chakra, which in turn will make the glands it supervises function better.

The energy center that oversees the neck region where the thyroid is located, is called *Vishuddhi*. The sound this chakra's vibration makes is 'ham', which is called its *beeja mantra* or seed sound. By repeating this mantra, you can stimulate the *Vishuddhi* into action. Similarly, the digestive organs such as the stomach, liver and pancreas are governed by the *Manipura Chakra* whose core sound is 'Ram'. You can meditate for 5 minutes on each of these two *chakra*s. The mantra can be simply repeated mentally or audibly. Rotating a rosary with the repetition is still better as that will make your mind more focussed.

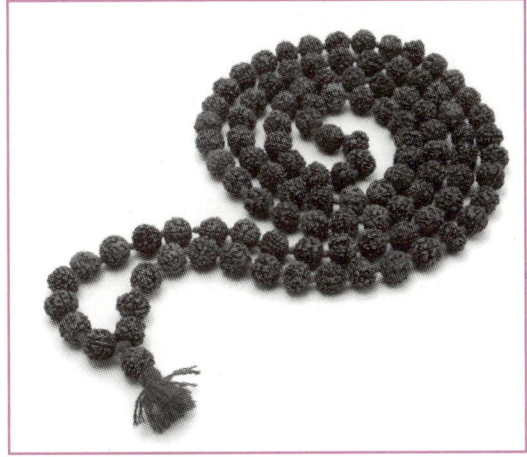

For the rosary, you can use rudraksh or choose a mixed one, i.e., *rudraksh* and colored stones. Each chakra has a specific colour using which the chakra can be influenced, while stones are known to affect the body in a positive way. So for *Vishuddhi,* whose colour is light blue, you can use blue stones with *rudraksh*. Similarly, yellow is the colour of Manipura, and hence for this chakra, the rosary should be *rudraksh* with yellow stones.

Technique

- Sit comfortably in any position.
- Relax your body.
- Breathe normally for a few minutes.
- Take the *mala* (yellow, if you are using the one with stones) in your right hand.
- Say 'Ram' and count a bead with your thumb (keep the index finger away from the *mala*).
- Repeat it for 5-6 minutes.
- Take a blue-stone mala and repeat the entire process with the mantra 'ham'.

Direct interaction

Around six trillion cells that make our body are living entities. They do everything that we humans do. Like us, they too eat, breathe, excrete, reproduce, communicate, and die. And they receive, understand and execute the orders coming from the brain precisely. If they are intelligent enough to understand the brain's intensions, they can understand it if they come from you too. When you give them some instructions with authority like the brain does, they will surely obey. It may take them a while to get used to orders coming from a different source, but eventually, they will respond if you are persistent.

Once a friend in her forties who was also a yoga practitioner was complaining about her increasing girth in spite of her food being the same as was in her thirties. I was meeting her briefly and had no time to check her *asanas* and *pranayamas* and add the relevant ones. So I told her to talk to her thyroid and taught her how to do it. Two years later, when I met her again, she had shed all the extra weight. When I commented on her trim body she proudly said, 'Yes, that too when I am eating more than I did earlier.' Then I asked her if she did it by speaking to her thyroid, and she looked back at me in wide-eyed surprise. She suddenly remembered the process that had helped her to reduce in six months. She had stopped doing that after she achieved her target, and had completely forgotten about it.

The best time to interact with the body's organs is immediately after *Yoganidra* or meditation when they are completely relaxed. Just stroke the area gently and repeat your order firmly in your mind. You can ask the thyroid to speed up the metabolism, the waist to be trimmer or the stomach to be satisfied with less food, while creating and holding a mental picture of what you want.

10 Tackling Depression

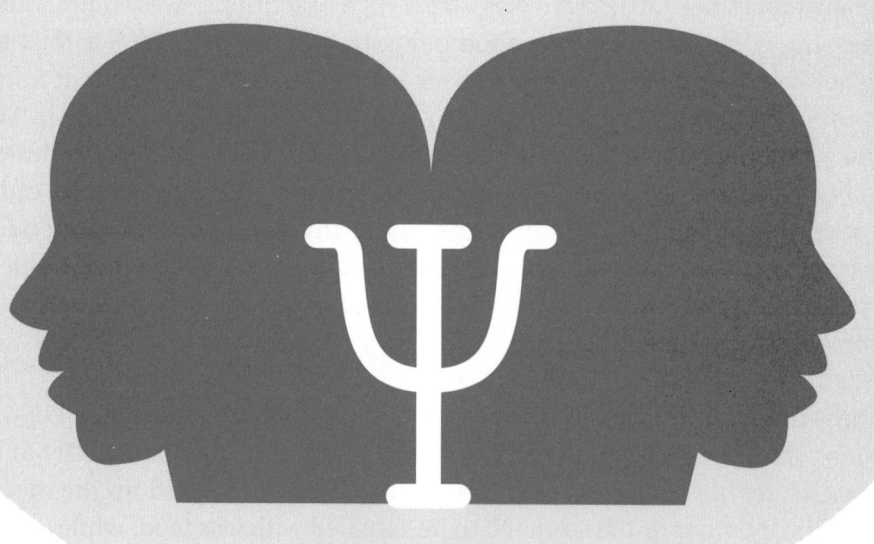

Tackling Depression

Depression has become quite common in today's world. Young or old, nobody is spared. Even school children are getting affected by this malady. And depression is one of the major causes of weight gain. It is mainly because depressed people develop a tendency to overeat, and that too all the wrong foods such as potato chips, chocolates, ice creams and the likes. Even though they are fully aware of the consequences of their actions, they just cannot help it. In depression, the urge to eat fattening food is too strong, and the will to resist it is too weak. To make matters worse, the affected people lack the zeal to exercise. Apart from not having the desire to do any physical activities, they simply don't have the energy to make the effort, as fatigue and lethargy are common symptoms of depression. Therefore, if this problem exists in an overweight person, it has to first sorted out.

The cause of depression can be anything from chronic stress, prolonged unhappiness, ill health, imbalance of hormones especially estrogen, birth control pills, and nutritional deficiencies of iron, potassium, tryptophan, manganese and vitamin B-complex, especially B12.

Conventionally, depression is treated with anti-depressant drugs or electric shock, which have many unpleasant side effects besides giving temporary and partial relief. Yoga with the right diet is the most effective method to counter this condition.

Yoga aims to remove the stress first. Although normal meditation and *Yoganidra* are generally used for the de-stressing, in depression, they can be counterproductive. Many depressive people have done them to cure their affliction and have ended up worsening it. It is because, the mind of depressive people is introverted and needs to be externalized whereas meditation and *Yoganidra* call for its internalization. Therefore, special kinds of meditations should be done in this condition. *Kirtan* (devotional music), *tratak*, and Om chanting are the best for them as these de-stressors take the mind out.

In addition to the mental yoga, relevant *asana*s and *pranayama* have to be practised to strengthen the nerves and normalize hormone secretion. For that purpose, the following *asana*s should be added to the slimming ones.

Apart from the Yogic regime, exposure to sunlight is essential for people suffering from depression. Because calcium, whose deficiency can cause this problem, is absorbed into the system only in the presence of Vitamin D, and it is sunlight that makes the body produce this vitamin. Vitamin D is not adequate in food sources.

SHASHANKASANA

Technique

- Sit with legs folded under you.
- Inhaling, raise your hands up.
- Exhaling, and moving the straight arms with the body, bend forward to keep the forehead on the ground.
- Hold the posture for a few seconds.
- Inhaling, straighten up to the arms raised position.
- Repeat 10 times.
- Lie down in *Shavasana* for 10 breaths.

CAUTION: Do not do this if you suffer from vertigo, slipped disc and cervical spondylitis.

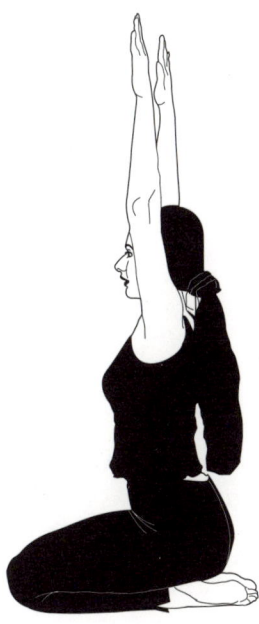

Shashakasana (static)

- Practise as above, but do it only once, and remain relaxed in the final position for 5 minutes, breathing normally.

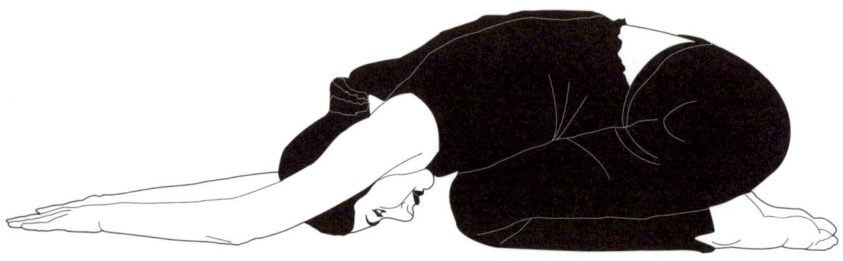

Important: The forehead must rest on the ground and not hang. If necessary, you may place a few books under the forehead.

CAUTION: Do not do this if you suffer from vertigo and slipped disc.

Bhumi Pada Mastakasana

- Sit with the legs folded under you.
- Placing the hands in front and away from you, lift the body up.
- Lower your head to place it on the ground in between the hands.

- Lift your hips and straighten the legs with the heels together and toes apart.
- Hold the hands behind and lift the toes.
- Breathing normally, hold the posture for as long as comfortable.
- Return to the starting position and place your forehead on the ground to rest for a few seconds.
- Lie down in *Shavasana* for 10 breaths.
- Starting with 1 round you can go up to 3 rounds.

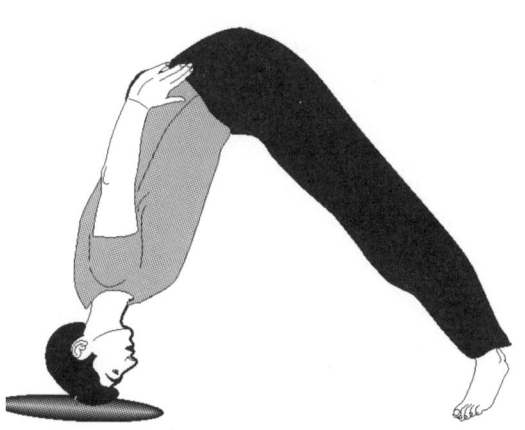

CAUTION: *Do not do this if your suffer from heart ailments, including high blood-pressure, any inflammation or infection in the head area, vertigo, severe eyesight problem, severe asthma, weak back, especially the neck, and when the blood is toxic.*

Shashankasana and *Bhumi Pada Mastakasana* bring more blood to the brain and improve the health of the nervous system.

Eka Pada Pranamasana

- Stand on the left leg with hands folded in front and the right foot on the left thigh, just above the knee.
- Look straight ahead and breathe deeply 20 times.
- Repeat on the right leg.

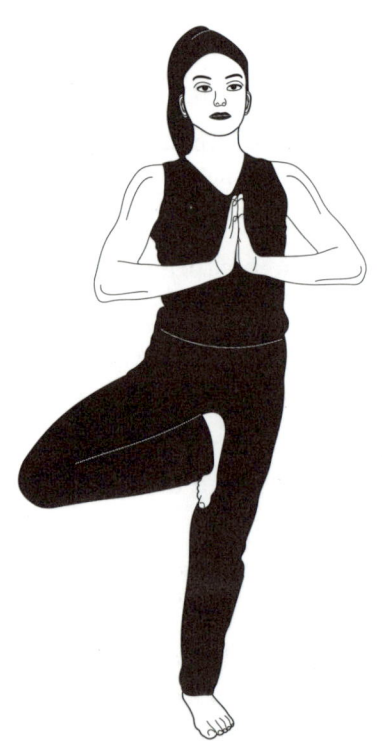

Natavara

- Stand on the left leg.
- Crossover the right leg to the left and place the right ankle a little above the left ankle with the toes pointing down.
- Join the thumbs with the middle fingers of the respective hands.
- Keep hands on the right side of the face separated by about 6 inches and away from the lips by 3.4 inches.

- Look straight ahead and breathe deeply 20 times.
- Repeat on the other side.

Eka pada pranamasana and Natavar also strengthen the nerves.

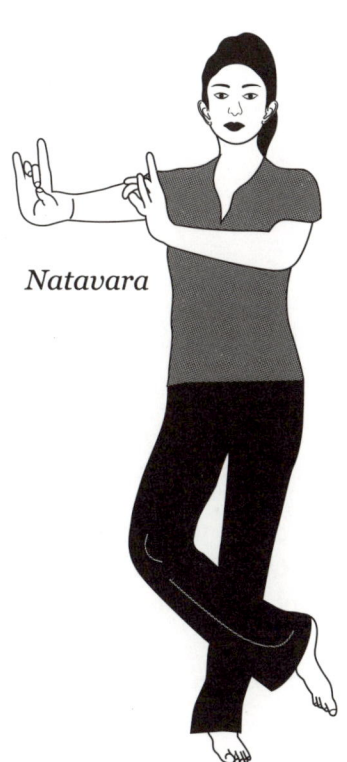

Natavara

CHAKRASANA

- Lie down on your back.
- Bend legs and place feet beside the hips.
- Place hands beside the neck with fingers pointing towards the body.
- Lift first the pelvic, then the shoulder and lastly the head as high as possible to form an arch.
- Breathe normally.
- Hold the posture for 10.20 breaths.
- While coming down, first put the head gently on the ground, roll it, then the shoulder and lastly the hip.

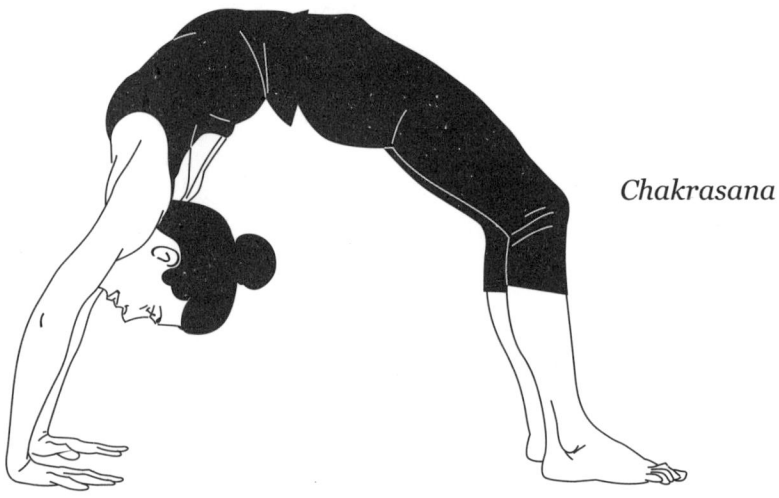

Chakrasana

CAUTION: *Do not do this if you suffer from heart ailments, high blood-pressure, stomach ulcer, hernia, weak wrist spinal problems and when the blood is toxic.*

Chakrasana improves the glandular functions.

Tratak

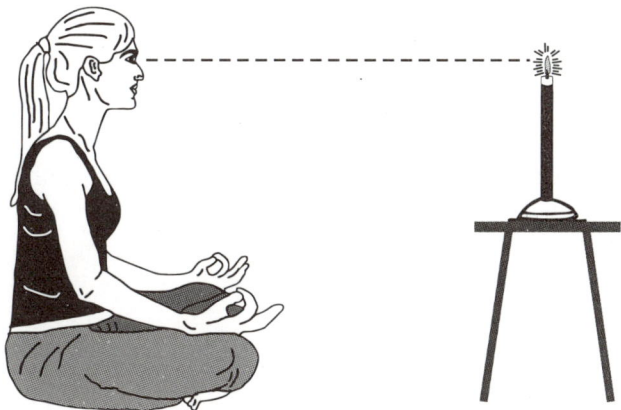

(Although Tratak is seen to be beneficial, it should be introduced after a week or so with caution and its effect observed. If the condition aggravates, it should be discontinued.)

Important: If there is no marked improvement within a month, conventional medication should be taken simultaneously till required.

Diet of a depressed person must be looked into and adjusted as required. Spinach, peas, broccoli, asparagus, milk, cheese and egg should be taken for folic acid and Vitamin B12, whose deficiencies can cause depression. Copper and lead deposit in the system that can lead to this problem are effectively removed by selenium, which is found in wheat germ, onion, tuna, nuts and seeds. Banana is also necessary for tryptophan that converts to serotonin, the feel good hormone. Nutmeg should also be taken daily as it works on the cerebral cortex and produces a euphoric feeling.

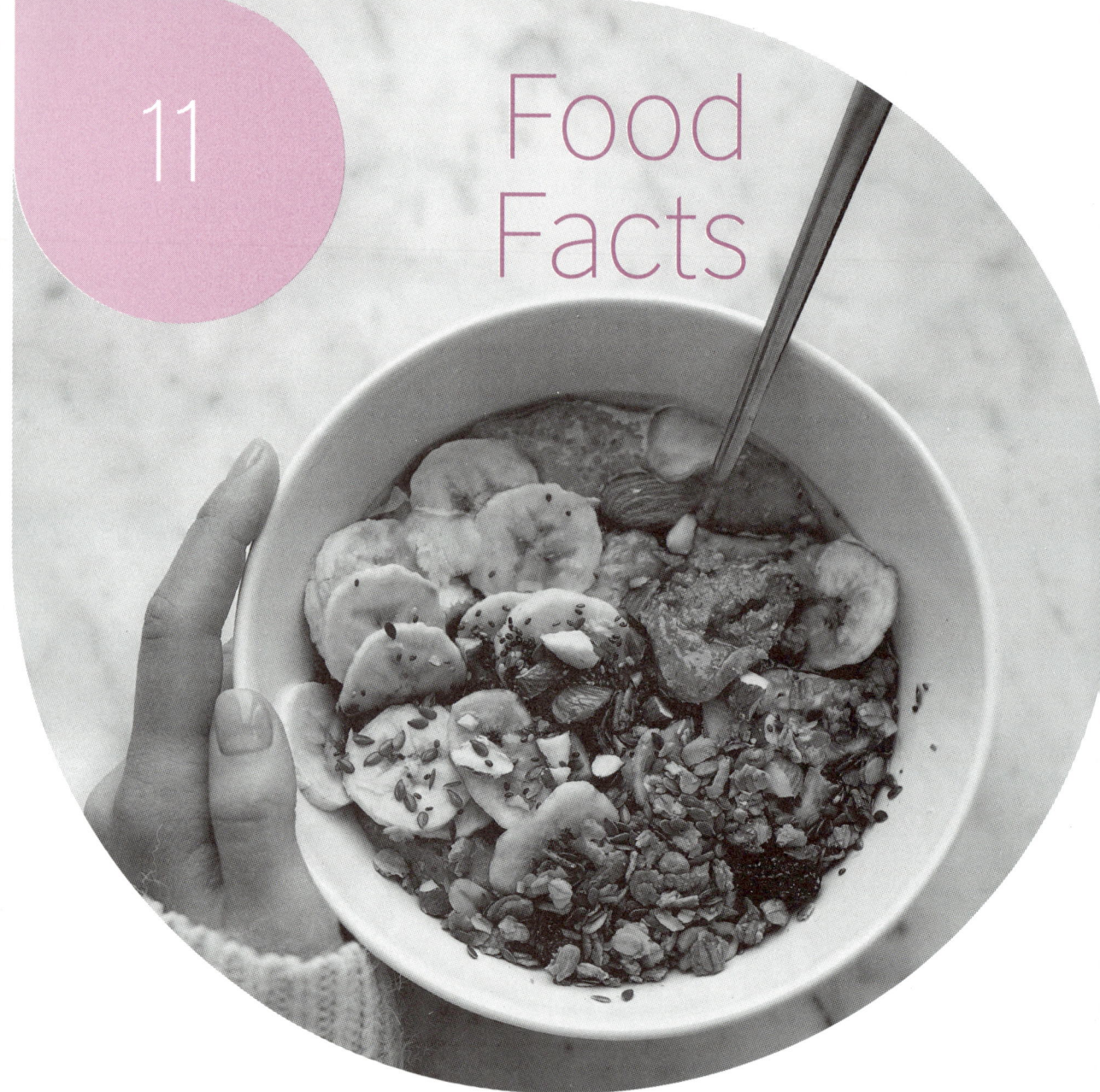

11 Food Facts

Food Facts

You are what you eat. This is a universal truth. Yoga too believes in it. That is why it calls the physical body an 'Annamaya sharira' meaning the body of food. Every tissue, which is the building block of our body, is made and renewed from food only. But not all of them need the same kind of food. Apart from certain common nutrients such as proteins, fats and carbohydrates, every body part comprising a group of tissues needs specific nutrients to live and function properly. For example, the bones can't do without calcium while for the blood it is iron, and for the nerves it is Vitamin B. Similarly, for the thyroid it is iodine.

Iodine is found in every food coming from the sea. For people who do not take sea food, there is iodized salt. Vegetarians who have given up sea salt or have switched over to rock salt do not have the required amount of iodine in their system for the thyroid to work efficiently. And without sufficient thyroxin, the metabolism has to slow down leading to weight gain.

It is not just iodine that we need to take to boost our metabolism, but also the nutrients needed by the other body parts, because all the glands and organs are interrelated and interdependent. The thyroid health may not be perfect when some other gland and organ is starving. Therefore, taking a well rounded diet is the priority for every weight watcher.

Calorie determination

When the calorie intake is more than the body's capacity to burn it, the extra calories are stored as fat. Even with healthy metabolism, there is a limit to one's capacity to utilize calories, and it varies from person to person. It depends on the individual's age, gender and activities. You can find out your body's rate of metabolism only by trials. Although you can do it any time, you get the most correct picture after guru shankha prakshyalan. With this *kriya*, it is normal for the appetite to increase and one generally takes a high calorie diet without putting on any weight. Start recording your total calorie intake as well as your weight every day. The appetite will gradually decline, so will the quantity of food. The day your weight increases slightly, remember the number of calories you had taken that day. A little less calories than that should be your daily requirement to maintain your body.

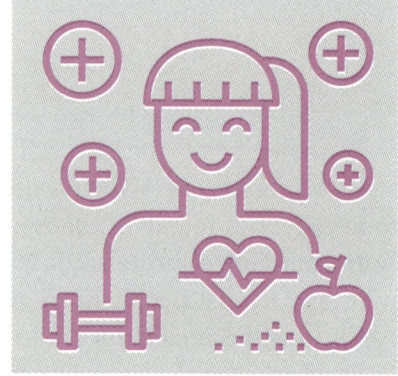

Once you have found out how much calorie you should consume, decide on their sources carefully. Because apart from calories, every food has certain other qualities too. It is necessary to know how the different sources work to choose the right ones for health and slimming. You also need to keep your individual taste in mind so that you will not feel deprived or else you may not be able to sustain it for long. So include everything that you like and adjust the calories otherwise. For example, if you like cakes, make it with whole wheat floor and jaggery and reduce your cereal in that meal. And include items that can be made without fat but are tasty.

Fat: Fat is the worst culprit for weight gain. 'Fat begets fat,' is a common saying and is very true. It is observed that the average Chinese people take 300 more calories per day than the Americans and yet are 25 per cent thinner. It is because fat constitutes 37 per cent of the total calories in the Americans' food while for the Chinese it is only around 6 to 14 per cent.

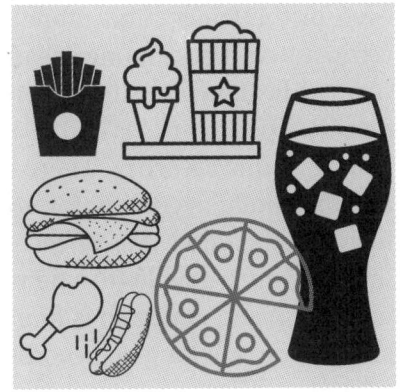

But, fat is essential to health. Some people completely eliminate fat from their diet for faster slimming, which is a dangerous practice. Our body needs fat for many of its functions. First, it is the medium for oil soluble Vitamins like A, D, E and K, and hence, in its absence, these vitamins cannot be absorbed into the system. Secondly, our nerves, including that of the brain, are made up of fat and need a continuous supply of it to remain healthy. And lastly, hormones, which regulate all our bodily functions are manufactured from cholesterol, a fat. Therefore, fat has to be taken every day to keep the body going. But all dietary fats are not the same. Some are good and some are harmful. Therefore, even the small percentage you need to take should be from the healthy sources.

There are basically two types of fats—saturated and unsaturated. Saturated fat is found in meat poultry and solid oil like palm oil, while various cooking oils are unsaturated. The latter one is further divided into polyunsaturated, which are liquid even in the fridge, and monounsaturated, which although thick are not hard when refrigerated. These monounsaturated fats are considered good for health as they lower the bad fat Low-density lipoprotein (LDL) in the body and raise the good one High-density lipoprotein (HDL). Fats of nuts such as olive, almond, walnut and peanut belong to this category. There is another type of fat called essential fatty acids, which are absolutely necessary for good health. They are Omega 3 and Omega 6. They too increase the good fats of the body. And good fats lead to better sugar and insulin metabolism, which in turn help in weight loss in the long run. Omega 3 is found mainly in oily fish and Omega 6 is found in seeds. As Omega 6 has a negative effect on weight, choose your cooking oil accordingly.

Sugar: The body's main fuel is glucose. When glucose comes to the blood from the digestive system, insulin is secreted by the pancreas. More the glucose in the blood, more is the insulin produced. This chemical pushes the glucose into the cells to be burnt to release energy. If the amount of glucose is more than the body's need for energy at a particular time, the surplus is converted into fat. Some food items, such as sugar have high glucose content which comes to the blood in a sudden surge and surpasses the

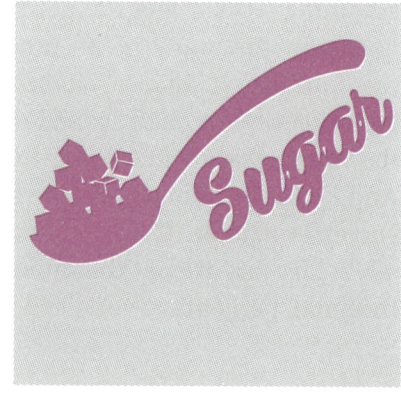

body's energy requirements at that moment. But when the glucose comes from cereals, its amount is not high and it is released into the blood at a slow and steady pace that matches the body's needs and is completely used up.

In a study, animals who were given sugar gained more weight and had more body fat than animals who did not take sugar, even though their total calorie intake of the day was identical. Therefore, do not consume too much calories from fat and sugar. It should not exceed 10-15 per cent of the total calorie consumption.

Carbohydrates: This is our main source of energy. Like fats, all carbohydrates are not the same with regards to their digestion or absorption time. Which means, they do not raise the blood glucose to the same level. Some release glucose slowly, which is completely utilized in the body's normal activities, while some release glucose too quickly leading to an excess in the blood than the body's need and the surplus is converted into fat. Another adverse effect of surplus glucose in the blood is the higher amount of insulin that was secreted, remains unutilized in the blood, exposing one to the risk of diabetes. Therefore, slow glucose releasing cereals should be preferred for health and a trim body. An example of such a cereal is ragi.

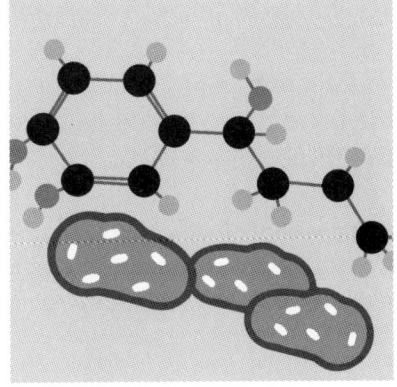

Most importantly, ensure that you take all the nutrients and at the right time. For example, Vitamin A gets depleted fast during stress, and hence, food rich in this vitamin should be taken in every meal. Similarly, Vitamin B, which is essential for the nerves, cannot be absorbed without Vitamin C and the body cannot store Vitamin C. Therefore, this vitamin also has to be taken in every meal.

Coconut is an important food for the thyroid and should be taken at least two three times a week.

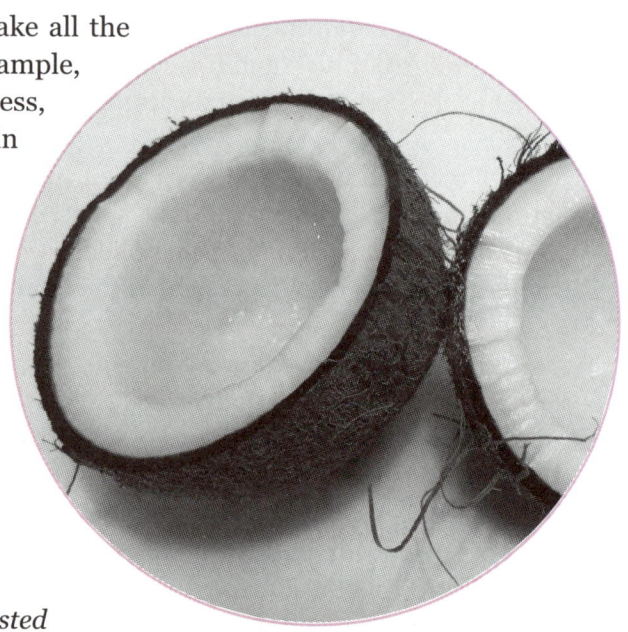

Some sample food charts containing all the nutrients. The quantity should be adjusted according to one's capacity to metabolize.

1. *Morning (every week-day when you are not doing Laghoo Shankha Prakshyalan)*

A glass of warm water with 1 tbs cider vinegar (3 calories) and 1 tbs honey (60 calories)

Breakfast	Noon	Lunch	Evening	Dinner
Poached egg (70 c) on toast (65 c)	A plateful of fruits (100 cal)	Rice ½ cup (100 c) and one roti medium (80c)	Tea (50 c)	Brown pasta with mushroom, broccoli 1 cup (100 c)
Sprouts 1 tbs (30 c) and almond chutney (20 c)		Daal ½ cup (50c)	Mixed nuts 1 tbs (50 c) and seeds such as pumpkin, flax etc. 1 tbs (45 c)	Salad with lettuce and lemon 1 cup (20 c)
One Date (20 c) and one fig (30 c)		Spinach ½ cup (12c)		Ragi pudding ½ cup (100 c)
Tea/coffee (50 c)		Vegetable curry that includes a yellow vegetable 1 cup (70 c)		
		Buttermilk 1/2 cup (50 c)		

2

Breakfast	Noon	Lunch	Evening	Dinner
Idli 3 (120 c)	Coconut water (45 c)	Rice ½ cup (100 c)	Nuts 1 tbs (50c) and seeds 1 tbs (45c)	Mushroom ½ cup (40c) on 1 brown toast (70c)
Sambar 1/2 cup (100c)		Roti 1 (80c)	Tea/coffee (50 c)	Salad with lemon dressing 1 cup (20 c)
Coconut chutney 1 tbs (50c)		Chicken ½ cup (50 c)		Mixed dry fruit dessert ½ cup (100c)
Rose hips 2 (1 c)		Mixed vegetable curry that includes green papaya 1 cup (70c)		
Tea/coffee (50c)		Green chutney 1 tbs (20 c)		
		Buttermilk ½ cup (50 c)		

3

Breakfast	Noon	Lunch	Evening	Dinner
Oats ½ cup (150 c) with one banana (100 c) one date (20c) one fig (30c) and milk (100c)	Vegetable juice that includes beetroot (50 c)	Rice 1/2 cup (100c)	Seeds and nuts (90c)	Sprout salad wrap with lemon squeezed in it 2 (200c)
Tea/coffee (50c)		One Roti (80c)	Tea/coffee (50c)	Apple bake ½ cup (70c)
		Fish ½ cup (100c)		
		Mixed vegetables curry of white pumpkin, squash, bottle gourd, and tomato 1 cup (80c)		
		Green chutney 1 tbs (20 c)		
		Buttermilk 1/2 cup (50c)		

HELPFUL TIPS

Eat half a grapefruit before every meal. According to a study conducted over 12 weeks on 100 obese people in America, the average weight loss among people who had this fruit was 4.5 kg while the group that did not lost only 225 gm. And a group who were given grapefruit juice to drink lost 1.5 kg.

Take 1/2 tsp cinnamon powder twice daily. It is seen to help control the blood sugar level which in turn prevents the body from storing fat.

Choose millets over your regular cereals. Millets are rich in fibre and the body burns up to 30 per cent more calories digesting fibres.

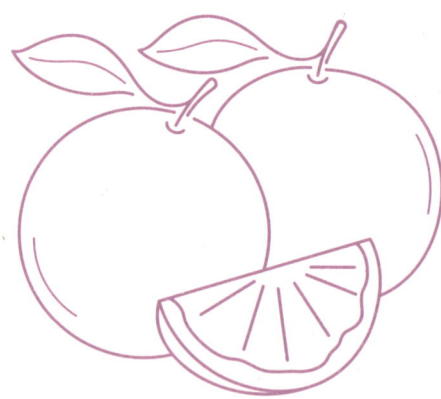

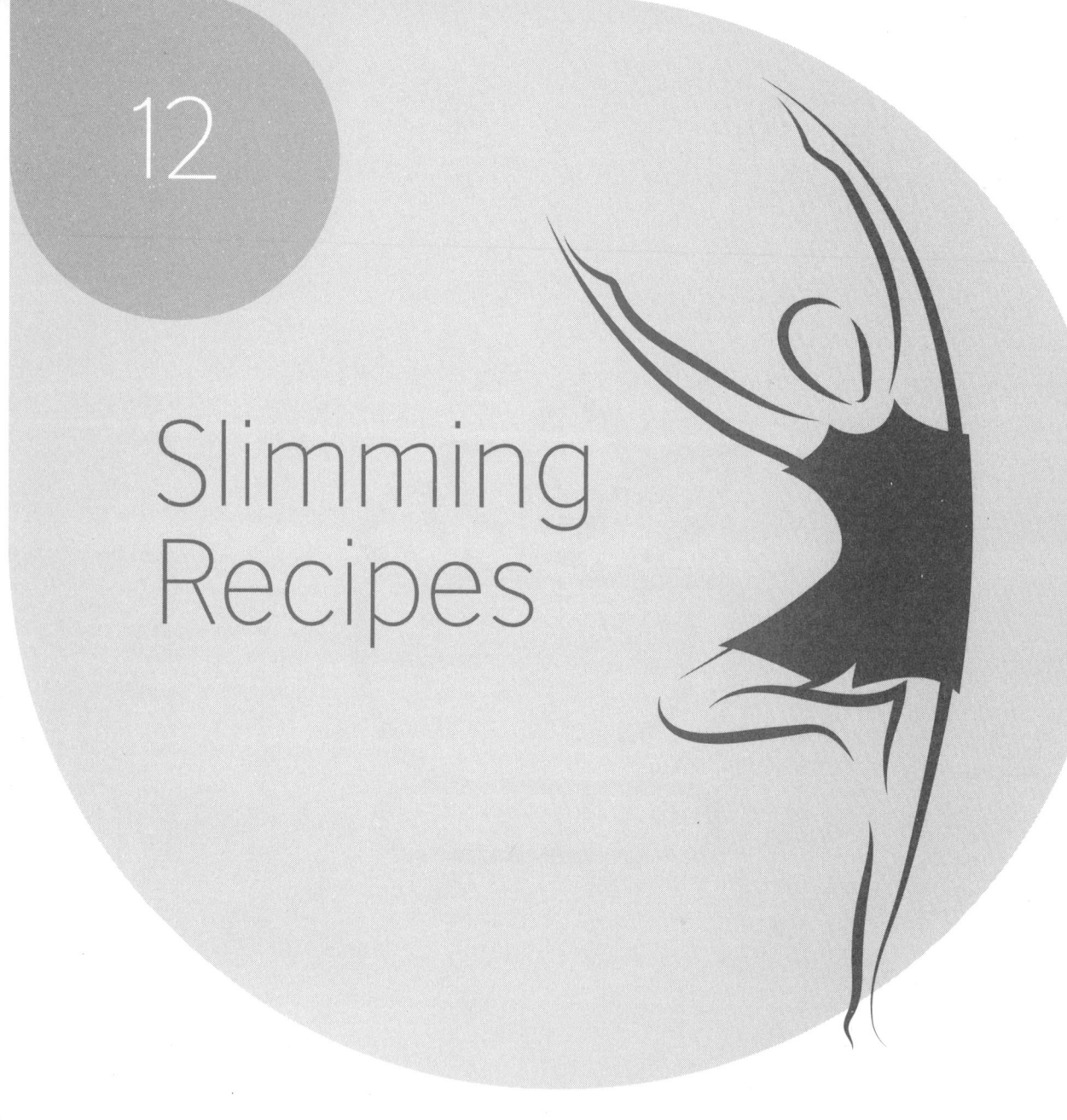

12
Slimming Recipes

Slimming Recipes

It is a general impression that slimming food is not tasty. There is absolutely no truth in it. Cooking is an art. Those who have mastered it can produce lip smacking items which are of low calorie.

Using some slimming ingredients such as mustard seeds help. It has been seen that 1 tsp of these seeds increase the metabolism of the body by 20-25 per cent for several hours after a meal. Other slimming spices are pepper and fennel. But mustard and pepper are acid producing. Therefore, if you are having an item with these spices, you should have other items with high alkaline levels to neutralize the acids. Also, as mustard is heavy on the stomach, it should be taken in the meals during the day and not at night when the digestive capacity is lower. People with acidity and arthritis should avoid it altogether.

Fish mustard

Ingredients

Fish	4 pieces	Tomato	1
Green chili	1	Onion	1/2
Garlic	6 cloves	Mustard seeds	2 tsp
Caraway seeds	¼ tsp	Turmeric	1/2 tsp
Oil	2 tsp	Salt to taste	
Water	1 cup	Coriander leaves for garnishing	

Method: Wash fish, rub salt and turmeric powder on it and keep aside. Grind the mustard seeds and garlic. Slice the onion. Chop the tomato. Heat oil in a pan and add the caraway seeds. When they crackle, split a green chilli and add it to the pan with the onion and fry till brown. Add the ground spice and tomato and fry for a minute. Put in the fish and fry a little. Pour water and simmer till done. Sprinkle chopped coriander leaves.

Steamed fish mustard

Ingredients

Fish	4 pieces	Mustard seeds	2 tsp
Khus khus	2 tsp	Coriander leaves	1 or 2 twigs
Mint leaves	1 or 2 twigs	Garlic	6 cloves
Green chilli	1	Turmeric	1/2 tsp
Oil	2 tsp	Lemon juice	1 tsp
Salt to taste			

Method: Wash fish and rub lemon, salt, oil and turmeric. Grind all the other ingredients together and mix with fish. Put the pieces in a banana or any edible leaf, wrap them well and steam for 7 minutes.

(These leaves have life and hence generate 'prana', which gets mixed with the food and benefits the system.)

Fish with tomato and celery

Ingredients

Fish	4 pieces	Tomato	4
Celery chopped	1/2 cup	Onion	½
Garlic	6 cloves	Ginger	1"
Green chili	1	Turmeric	1/2 tsp
Oil	2 tsp	Cumin seed powder	2 tsp
Chili powder	1/4 tsp	Water	1 cup
Salt to taste			

Method: Wash the fish and rub salt and turmeric on it. Heat oil in a *kadai* till smoking. Twirl the *kadai* to coat it's sides well with the oil. Spread the fish pieces one at a time so that they do not stick together. After 2-3 minutes when the lower part is golden, turn them over and fry the other side. Remove and keep aside. Blanch tomatoes and chop. Grate the ginger. Chop onion, garlic and green chili. Put all the chopped items, salt, chili powder and water in a pot and cook till soft. Puree it or leave it as it is. Add the fish and simmer for 5 minutes. Remove from fire. Dry roast cumin seed powder and sprinkle over it.

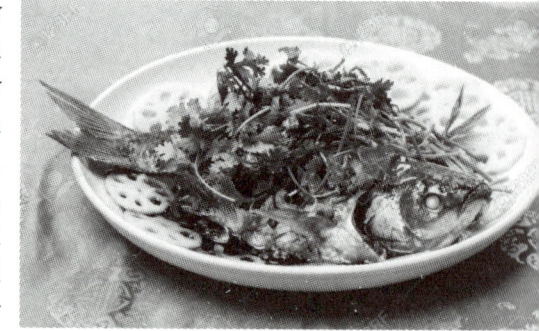

Baked salmon

Ingredients

Salmon	2 pieces	Garlic	8 cloves
Oil	2 tsp	Salt to taste	

Method: Grind garlic and mix with the oil and salt. Wash the fish and coat the pieces with the paste. Marinate for an hour and bake them for 5-6 minutes.

Chicken pepper

Ingredients

Chicken pieces	6	Oil	2 tsp
Freshly crushed pepper	1 tsp	Salt to taste	

Method: Wash and dry the chicken pieces. Heat oil and fry the chicken on high flame. When the raw smell disappears, add water, salt and pepper and cook till done.

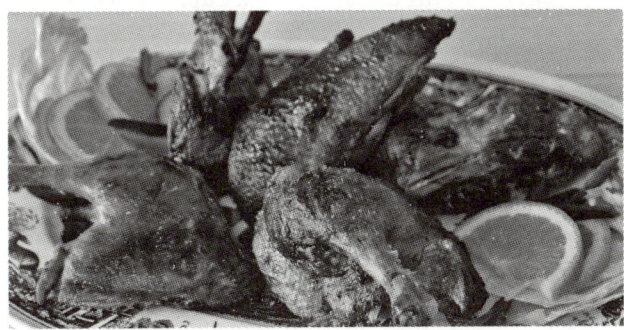

Chicken teriyaki

Ingredients

Chicken	6 pieces	Teriyaki sauce	4 tsp
Garlic	6 cloves	Honey	½ tsp
Pepper	a pinch		

Method: Wash the chicken. Mix it with all other ingredients and keep aside for an hour and grill till done.

Mustard cabbage

Ingredients

Cabbage shredded	2 cups	Tomato	1/2
Mustard seeds	2 tsp	Garlic	6 cloves
Green chili	1	Oil	2 tsp
Salt to taste			

Method: Grind mustard with garlic and chili and mix it with the cabbage. Put all the ingredients in a pot and cover it. Cook it on low flame. The vegetables should leave water enough to get cooked in it. In case it becomes dry, add a little water.

Mustard okra

Ingredients

Okra	1 dozen	Mustard seeds	2 tsp
Garlic	4 cloves	Tomato	1
Red chili	1	Fenugreek seeds	¼ tsp
Turmeric	½ tsp	Oil	2 tsp
Salt to taste		Water	¼ cup or even less

Method: Chop tomato. Grind mustard and garlic. Wash, dry and split the okra lengthwise. Heat oil. Add the chili and fenugreek seeds to it. When the crackling stops, add okra pieces with turmeric, and fry them for 3-4 minutes. Add tomato and salt and fry for another minute or two before adding the paste. Again fry for a minute or two. Pour in the water and simmer till cooked and the water has evaporated.

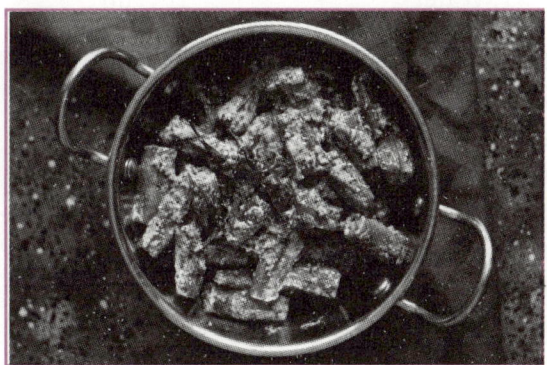

Mixed veg mustard

Ingredients

Green papaya diced	1/2 cup	Bottle gourd diced	½ cup
Brinjal diced	½ cup	Potato diced	1/2 cup
Mustard seeds	1 tsp	Garlic	6 cloves
Green chili	1	Oil	1 tsp
Mustard seed for tempering	¼ tsp	Salt to taste	
Water	1/3 cup		

Method: Cook vegetables with salt and water. Grind mustard seeds, garlic and chili. When the vegetables are cooked, add the ground spices. Simmer it for 3-4 minutes and remove from fire. Heat the oil and add the remaining mustard seeds. At the fag end of the crackling, add the vegetables and simmer for a minute.

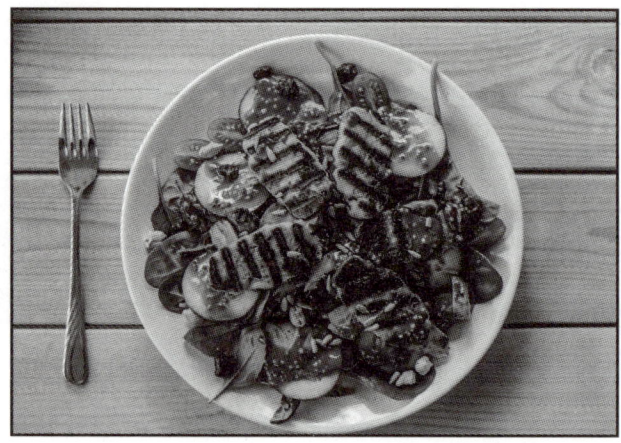

Another style

Ingredients

Potato	1	Brinjal	½
Pumpkin (half ripe)	3" piece	Green banana	1
Tomato	1	Mustard seeds	2 tsp
Cumin seeds	1 tsp	Garlic	6 cloves
Chili powder	¼ tsp	Turmeric	½ tsp
5 tempering spices (mustard, fenugreek, fennel, caraway, cumin)			½ tsp
Red chili	1	Salt to taste	
Water	1 cup		

Method: Halve the banana and soak it in water. Peel a potato and cut it lengthwise. Cut the pumpkin and eggplant in a similar manner. Peel the banana and cut it the same way. Cut tomato into big pieces. Grind mustard, cumin and garlic. Split the red chili. Cook all the vegetables except tomato with water salt and turmeric till done. Heat oil. Add the 5 spices and red chili. As the crackling reduces, add the ground spices and chili powder. Fry for 2–3 minutes. Pour in the cooked vegetables and simmer for 3–4 minutes.

Beans with fennel

Ingredients

Beans diced	1 cup	Oil	2 tsp
Fennel seed powder	1 tsp	Dry ginger powder	1/2 tsp
Pepper crushed	1/4 tsp	Asafoetida	a pinch
Salt	to taste	Water	1/2 cup

Method: Cook the beans with salt and water. Let the water evaporate completely. Remove from fire. Heat oil. Add the asafoetida. When nicely aromatic, add the beans and fry till the oil glistens. Add the powdered spices and fry for a minute.

Fruit dessert

Ingredients

Apple	1	Banana	1
Raisins	2 tsp	Cashew nuts	5 – 6
Sugar	2 tsp	Cinnamon powder	1/2 tsp

Method: Peel, core and cut the apple into thin wedges. Peel and slice banana. Spread the fruits in a baking dish, sprinkle sugar and cinnamon powder and bake. When half done sprinkle the nuts and raisins and bake till soft and slightly caramelized.

Apple bake

Ingredients

Apple	1 small	Molasses	1 tbs
Green cardamom	1	Coconut (scraped)	1 tbs
Salt	a pinch		

Method: Core the apple from the top. Powder the cardamom. Fill up the apple with all the ingredients and bake till soft.

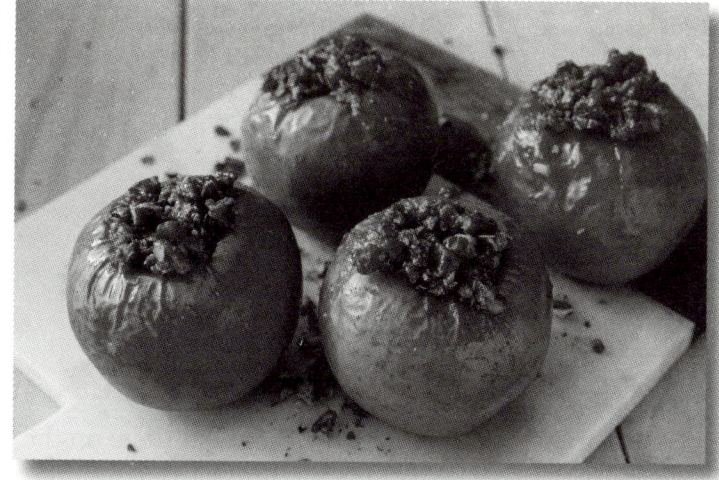

Dry fruit dessert

Ingredients

Dried figs	2	Dates	2
Dried apricot	2	Raisins	1 tsp
Apple	½	Cinnamon	1 big piece
Sugar	1-2 tsp	Water	½ cup

Method: Wash and cut the apple and figs. Stone apricot. Heat a pot and add sugar. Keep stirring for even caramelizing. When nicely brown, pour in the water. Add all other ingredients. Cook till the apple is soft and the water has evaporated.

Ragi pudding

Ingredients

Ragi powder	1/2 cup	Jaggery	a little less than ½ cup
Water	2½ cup		

Method: Mix all the ingredients and put them on the flame. Keep stirring and cook it for 10-15 minutes. When the mixture becomes a little translucent, remove it from the flame, cool and refrigerate it.

Sprout chutney

Ingredients

Green gram sprouts	½ cup	Almonds	20
Green chili	1	Extra virgin olive oil	1 tbs
Grated Coconut	1/2 cup	Amla or cider vinegar to taste	
Salt to taste			

Method: Add all the ingredients except the oil and vinegar in a mixi and make a smooth paste. Add the liquids and refrigerate.

Green Chutney

Ingredients

Coriander leaves	a large bunch	Mint leaves	a small bunch
Green chili	1	Salt	
Amla or cider to taste			

Method: Add all the ingredients except the vinegar in a mixi and make a smooth paste. Add the liquid and refrigerate.

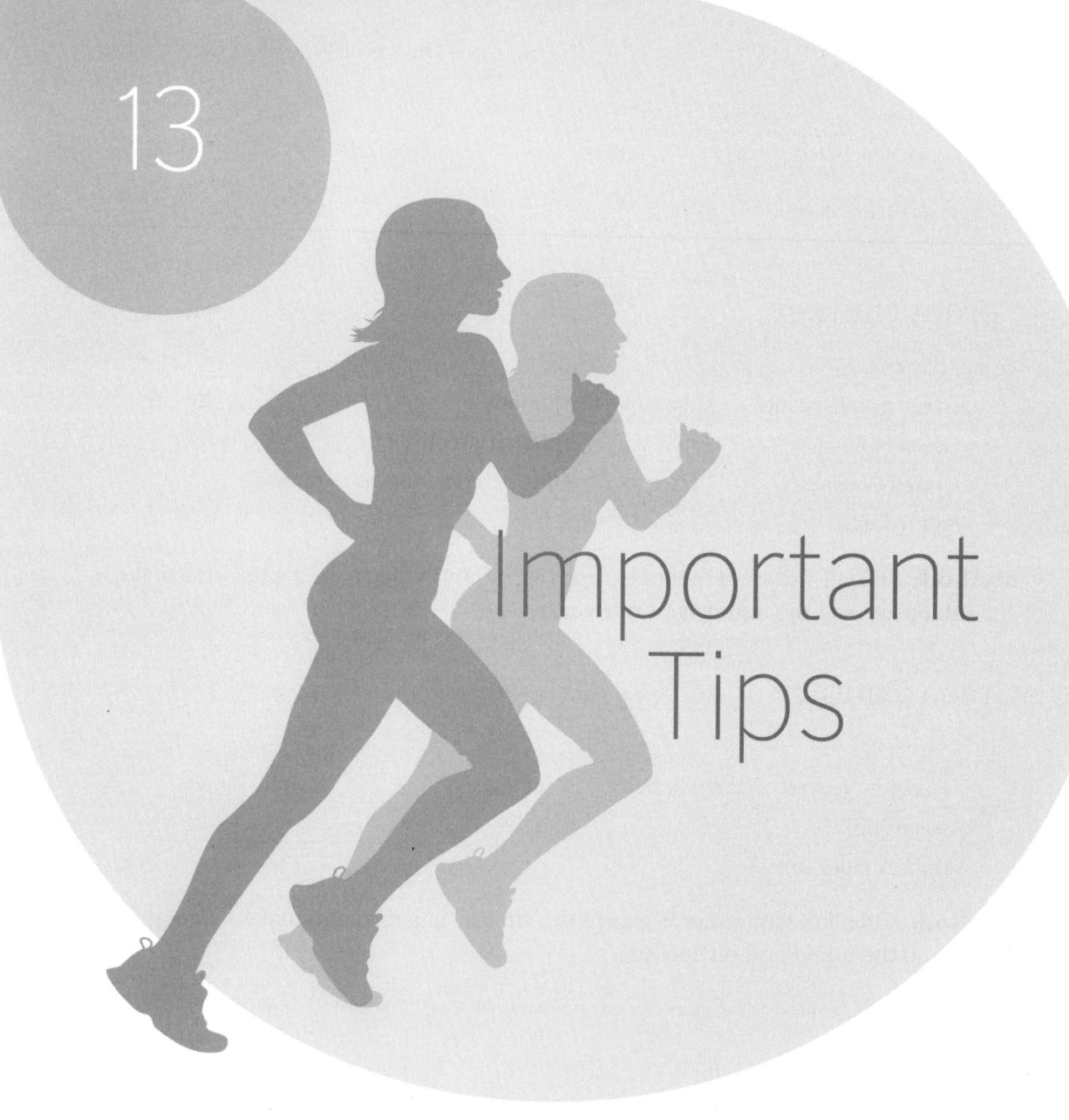

13

Important Tips

Important Tips

There is a misconception that doing an hour of yoga is sufficient to maintain good health. It is not so. It is necessary to adopt a balanced lifestyle to be truly healthy.

When I first gained some weight before I had become obese, and was unable to shed it with normal exercises, I asked my mother what I should do. Her simple reply was, "Eat what I eat and do what I do." I reflected on her words. She was a slim woman who had never ever put on any weight in spite of eating many hearty meals a day. Although her food was the typical Odia—simply steamed or boiled, rarely fried.

Till then, my diet was high-calorie *puris*, *parathas*, curries with oil floating on them, and all kinds of sweets. I had never fancied Odia food. My taste buds had become too spoilt to like the blandness. But what choice did I have? I was desperate to get back into my former shape. So I agreed to give it a try. Initially I had to force the food down my throat. But after a while, surprisingly, I started enjoying it. It was such a relief! One problem was solved.

It was the second part of my mother's advice that I found was the bigger problem. She was mobile all the time while I was just the opposite. She would cook, do most of the household chores and when she was not doing either, she would just walk round the house, inspecting what needed to be done or stroll in the garden. Whereas for me, it was my a book in bed which she did not allow anymore. She saw to it that I didn't remain idle even for a moment. First, she made me sweep the floor and do the dusting even though the maid would have already finished doing that. Thereafter, every time she would see me in bed, she would nag me to get up and take a thousand steps. I would grumble but would have to do it. And it paid off! I started losing weight quickly. The combination of right food and continuous movement really does wonders to the body.

Unfortunately, in today's world with remote controls, escalators and elevators, people hardly move. Except for the health conscious, for whom walking is a part of their exercise regime, others might not be taking even a few hundred steps in the whole day. Even for the latter category, walking once a day may not help if they are sitting rest of the time. Because sitting for long hours stiffens the blood vessels, which not only puts the cardiovascular system at a great risk but also the blood supply to all other body tissues is adversely affected. In such a condition, the thyroid cannot become super efficient. Even yoga may not rectify the condition as the negative effect of a static body can overtake yoga's good effects.

Therefore, to maintain good health of any body part, it is necessary to move it, and walking is the best way to do that. In any case walking is essential in life. It is the most basic of all activities. Nobody teaches a baby how to walk. It does it instinctively. Not only that, it spends most of its waking time walking. And anything that nature intends humans to do is necessary for their survival and good health. Primitive man did not do yoga to remain fit. All he did was walked and remained active. Even fifty years ago, people walked a lot. They went to their destinations—schools, colleges, offices, or market—on foot.

Apart from many proven health benefits, walking also is a mood lifter. In a British study, office workers reported increased enthusiasm and relaxation after thirty minutes of lunch-break walk.

Still better result is achieved by walking outdoor surrounded by trees. That way, more oxygen and *prana* get into the system while the beauty and colours of the nature relax and soothe the nerves. Furthermore, some scientists believe that the phytoncides molecules secreted by trees that are absorbed by the skin and respiratory systems have many health benefits. It strengthens the immune system, reduces stress level, lowers blood pressure and lifts depression. Ayurveda recommends walking bare feet on grass for enhanced effect. In Japan, some artificial forests have been created for people to walk in them. It is known as forest therapy, which involves strolling slowly in the woods, barefoot and hug the trees. They also call it 'shinrin–yoku', meaning forest breathing.

Therefore, for physical and mental health and for a trim body, make it a point to walk-not only a brisk long walk of thirty-forty minutes daily but also for a few minutes every hour.

Deep Breathing

As has been earlier said, more of *prana* in our system, better is our health. This vital force gets into the body mainly with the breath. But when people's mind is occupied with planning, calculating and worrying, and during such conditions, the breathing automatically becomes shallow that decreases the inflow of *prana* into the body. As it is, the city air does not have much of this energy. Mountain air has been measured to have 5,000 units of it per 300 cubic feet against 50 units in a city room. Therefore, we need to do a conscious effort to absorb more of it and the only way to that is to breathe deeply every now and then.

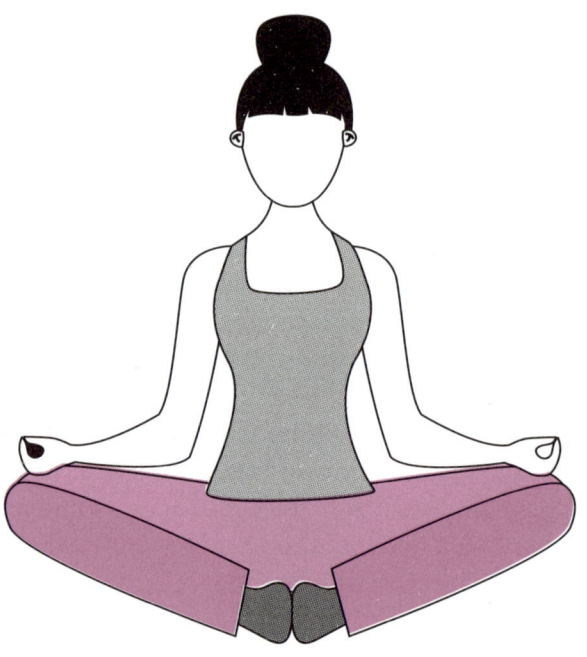

Massage

Massage is a part of traditional living. In India, it starts with the day a baby is born. Both the newborn and its new mother are massaged daily for twenty-one days minimum. Old people too get it done regularly. And it is a part of Ayurvedic treatment for many maladies. Weight loss is one of them.

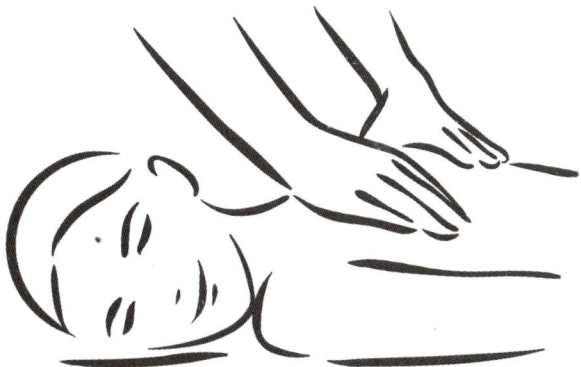

When one starts losing weight fast, the skin, which was stretched to hold the fat can sag and look ugly. Massage can prevent that. At the same time, it can give many other health benefits. According to Mayo Clinic, massage is helpful for anxiety, digestive disorders, fibromyalgia, headaches, insomnia, soft tissue strain, sports injury and more.

Today, massage has become very popular all over the world and many types of massages are available. Although it is more pleasant and convenient to get it done by somebody else, one can also do it on one's own. In my experience, it is not much less effective, especially for the purpose of slimming. I have seen the following methods work well.

Technique:

- Apply some talcum powder on the body part to be massaged.
- Start with very mild strokes, then move to stronger strokes.
- Then knead and pinch the muscles.
- On the thighs, grasp a portion with both hands and move the hands in opposite directions so that the movement make the shape of an 'S'.
- Again, use strokes but from stronger to milder to the mildest.

All massage should be done towards the heart.

A sample daily routine

Morning

- Either *Laghoo Shankha Prakshyalan* or a long walk in the sun.
- 15 minutes of rest.
- *Asanas* and *pranayamas*.

Evening

- Mantra meditation (can be done while returning from work provided you are not driving).

Bedtime

Tratak

Yoganidra. (It can be followed by direct interaction if you are not asleep by then. Otherwise, practise it after meditation.)

Meditation

Dinner